RENAL DIET COOKBOOK

PROTECT

YOUR

KIDNEYS

Delicious Recipes To Maintain A Healthy and Functioning Kidneys

LANEY BENDER

from the Publisher. All additional right reserved.

The information in the following pages is broadly considered to be a truthful and accurate account of facts and as such any inattention, use or misuse of the information in question by the reader will render any resulting actions solely under their purview. There are no scenarios in which the publisher or the original author of this work can be in any fashion deemed liable for any hardship or damages that may befall them after undertaking information described herein.

Additionally, the information in the following pages is intended only for informational purposes and should thus be thought of as universal. As befitting its nature, it is presented without assurance regarding its prolonged validity or interim quality. Trademarks that are mentioned are done without written consent and can in no way be considered an endorsement from the trademark holder.

Table of Contents

PART I 12

Pumpkin Pancakes 14

Pasta Salad 16

Broccoli and Apple Salad 17

Pineapple Frangelico Sorbet 19

Egg Muffins 20

Linguine With Broccoli, Chickpeas, and Ricotta 22

Ground Beef Soup 25

Apple Oatmeal Crisp 26

Chapter 2: Weekend Recipes for Renal Diet 27

Hawaiian Chicken Salad Sandwich 27

Apple Puffs 28

Creamy Orzo and Vegetables 30

Minestrone Soup 32

Frosted Grapes 34

Yogurt and Fruit Salad 35

Beet and Apple Juice Blend 37

Baked Turkey Spring Rolls 38

Crab-Stuffed Celery Logs 40

Couscous Salad 41

Chapter 3: One-Week Meal Plan 43

Chapter 4: Avoiding Dialysis and Taking the Right Supplements 46

PART II 50

Chapter 1: Introduction to the Low FODMAP diet 51

Getting Started 52

What is IBS? 52

Who is the diet for? 53

History of the low FODMAP diet 55

What does FODMAP stand for? 55

Sources of Fructans 57

Sources of Galactans 57

Sources of Polyols 58

Effectiveness and Risks of the low FODMAP diet 58

Chapter 2: Benefits of the Low FODMAP diet 60

Benefits of a Grain Free Diet 62

Chapter 3: Starting the Low FODMAP diet 66

Getting Diagnosed with IBS and FODMAP Tests 66

Medical Tests for IBS 68

Breaking down FODMAPS 69

Fermentable 69

Oligo-Saccharies 70

Di-Saccharies 70

Mono-Saccharides 70

And Polyols 71

The Elimination Phase 71

The Reintroduction Phase 72

Maintenance Phase 73

Low FODMAP Diet with Vegan/Vegetarian Diet 74

Low FODMAP Diet and Diabetes 75

Low FODMAP Diet for Children 76

Exercise on the Low FODMAP Diet 78

Reasons the Diet May Not Be Working 79

Chapter 4: Low FODMAP diet foods 82

Reading and Understanding Nutrition Fact Label 82

Chapter 5: Low FODMAP Diet Meal plan 96

Low FODMAP Breakfast Recipes: 96

Small Banana Pancakes 96

Ingredients 96

Instructions 97

Roasted Sausage and Vegetable Breakfast Casserole 98

Ingredients 98

Instructions 98

Blueberry Low FODMAP Smoothie 100

Ingredients: 100

Instructions: 100

Banana and Oats FODMAP Breakfast Smoothie 101

Ingredients 101

Instructions 101

Blueberry, Banana, and Peanut Butter Breakfast Smoothie 102

Ingredients 102

Instructions: 102

Kale, Ginger, and Pineapple Breakfast Smoothie 103

Ingredients: 103

Instructions: 103

Strawberry and Banana Breakfast Smoothie 104

Ingredients: 104

Instructions:..104

Low FODMAP Soups and Salads: 105

Apple, Carrot, and Kale Salad 105

Ingredients: 105

Instructions:..105

Green Bean, Tomato, and Chicken Salad 106

Ingredients: 106

Instructions:..106

Tuna Salad Low FODMAP Style.......................................107

Ingredients 107

Instructions..107

Low FODMAP Pumpkin Soup..108

Ingredients 108

Instructions..109

Quinoa and Turkey Meatball Soup 110

Ingredients: 110

Instructions:..110

Mixed Vegetable, Bean and Pasta Soup 111

Ingredients: 111

Instructions:..112

Vegan Options: 113

Low FODMAP Coconut and Banana Breakfast Cookie.........113

Ingredients: 113

Instructions:..114

Lemon and Garlic Roasted Zucchini.................................115

Ingredients: 115

Instructions: 115

Rainbow Low FODMAP Slaw 116

Ingredients: 116

Ingredients: 116

Vegan Roasted Red Pepper Farfalle 117

Ingredients: 117

Instructions: 117

Breakfast Meal Plan Ideas: 118

Lunch Meal Plan Ideas: 118

Dinner Meal Plan Ideas: 119

14- Day Meal Plan 120

Week One: 120

Week Two: 121

Vegan 7-Day Meal Plan 122

Chapter 6: Low FODMAP diet tips and tricks for success 123

Chapter 7: Low FODMAP diet FAQ 127

PART III 130

Chapter 1: How to Reset Your Body? 131

Chapter 2: Science Behind Metabolism Reset 133

Chapter 3: Recipes for Smoothies and Salads 135

Green Smoothie 135

Strawberry Banana Smoothie 136

Salmon Citrus Salad 137

Chapter 4: Quick and Easy Breakfast and Main Course Recipes 139

Quinoa Salad 139

Herb and Goat Cheese Omelet 141

Mediterranean Cod 143

Grilled Chicken and Veggies...145

Stuffed Peppers 148

Brussels Sprouts With Honey Mustard Chicken.......................151

Quinoa Stuffed Chicken 153

Kale and Sweet Potato Frittata.......................................155

Walnut, Ginger, and Pineapple Oatmeal.............................156

One-Pot Chicken Soup..160

Chocolate Pomegranate Truffles.....................................162

PART IV.. 163

Chapter 1: Tasty Breakfast Options 164

French Crepe 164

Chapter 2: Delicious Salads... 168

Traditional French Country Salad With Lemon Dijon Vinaigrette 168

Chapter 3: Soup 170

Classic French Onion Bistro Soup 170

Fresh French Pea Soup..172

Green Vegetable Soup 174

Chapter 4: Beef Options... 176

Beef Bourguignon - Slow-Cooked 176

Entrecote Steak With Red Wine Sauce 179

Pan-Seared Steak au Poivre..181

Steak Diane..183

Chapter 5: Other Delicious French Classics 185

French Ham & Grilled Cheese Sandwich - Croque Monsieur..............185

Pork Chops With Mustard Sauce 187

Provencal Chicken Casserole 189

White Wine Coq Au Vin.. 190

PART V 192

Chapter 1: Soup...193

Hot & Sour Soup 193

Wonton Soup 195

Chapter 2: Seafood...197

Honey Walnut Shrimp 197

Steamed Fish 199

Stir-Fried Shrimp & Scallions 201

Chapter 3: Poultry..202

Kung Pao Chicken - Keto-Friendly...................................... 203

Orange Chicken... 206

Chapter 4: Pork..209

Chinese Pork BBQ (Char Siu).. 209

Chinese Pork Dumplings... 211

Chop Suey 213

Easy Moo Shu Pork.. 215

Peking Pork Chops - Slow-Cooked 217

Chapter 5: Other Chinese Dishes.....................................219

Crispy Tofu With Sweet & Sour Sauce................................. 219

Shiitake & Scallion Lo Mein 222

PART I

Chapter 1:

Easy Recipes for Managing Kidney Problems

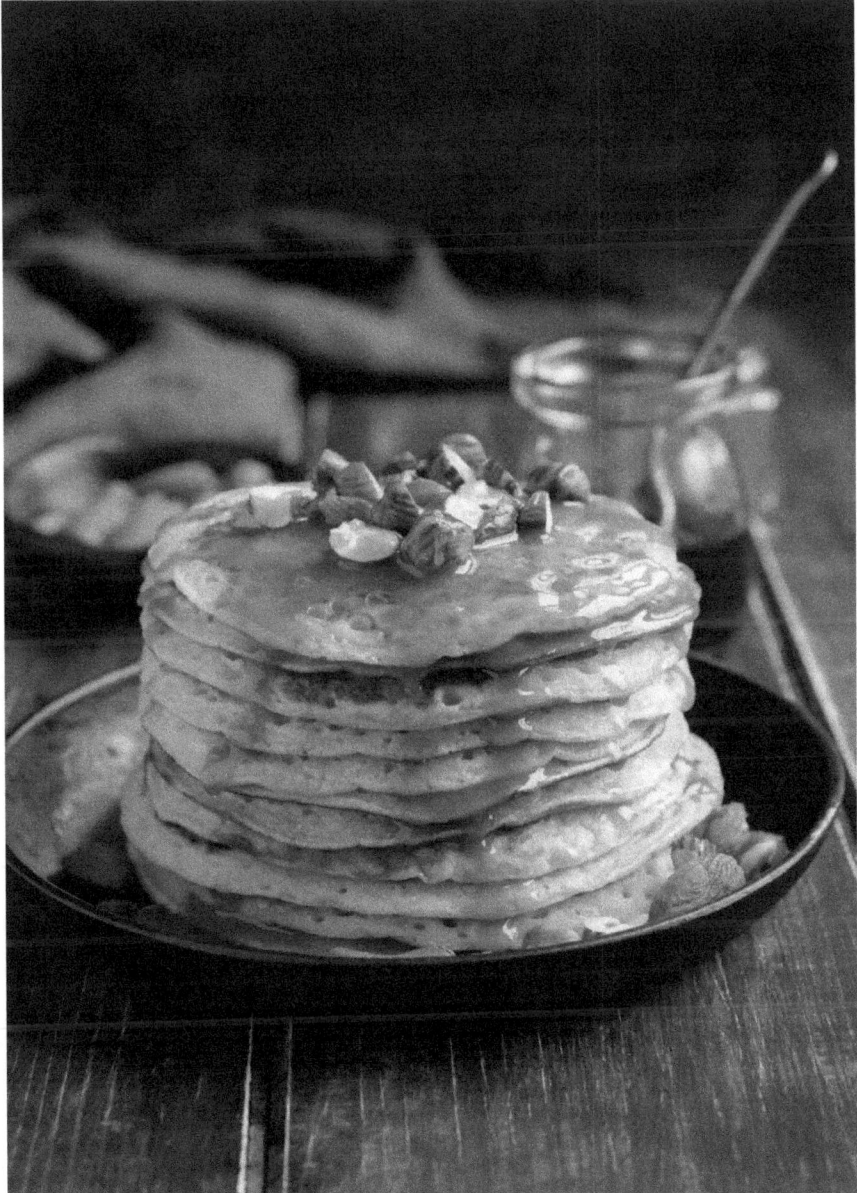

Pumpkin Pancakes

Total Prep & Cooking Time: 40 minutes

Yields: 2 servings

Nutrition Facts: Calories: 183 | Carbs: 39g | Protein: 5.4g | Fat: 1.2g | Sodium: 130mg

Ingredients:

- Two egg whites

- Two tsps. of pumpkin pie spice

- One tsp. of baking powder

- One tbsp. of brown sugar

- Three packets of Stevia

- 1.25 cups of all-purpose flour

- Two cups each of

  o Rice milk

  o Salt-free pumpkin puree

Method:

1. Start by mixing all the dry ingredients together in a bowl – baking powder, Stevia, sugar, flour, and pumpkin pie spice.

2. Now, take another bowl and, in it, mix the rice milk and pumpkin puree thoroughly.

3. In another bowl, form stiff peaks by whipping egg whites.

4. Take the mixture of dry ingredients and add them to the wet ingredients. Blend them in. Once you get a smooth mixture, add the egg whites, and whip them.

5. Grill the mixture on an oiled griddle on medium flame.

6. When you notice bubbles forming on the pancakes, you have to flip them.

7. Cook both sides of the pancakes evenly so that they turn golden brown.

Pasta Salad

Total Prep & Cooking Time: 50 minutes

Yields: 4 servings (half a cup each serving)

Nutrition Facts: Calories: 69 | Carbs: 12.5g | Protein: 2.5g | Fat: 1.3g | Sodium: 72mg

Ingredients:

- A quarter cup of olives (sliced after being pitted)
- One cup of chopped cauliflower
- Two cups of fusilli pasta (cooked)
- Half a unit each of
  - Green bell pepper (sliced)
  - Red onion (chopped)
  - Tomato (small-sized, diced)

Method:

1. Start by cooking the pasta, and for that, you have to follow the directions as mentioned on the package.

2. Now, drain the pasta. Add all the vegetables.

3. Choose any dressing of your choice, but it has to be low-fat. Toss the pasta and the veggies in the dressing.

4.   Serve and enjoy!

Broccoli and Apple Salad

Total Prep & Cooking Time: 15 minutes

Yields: 8 servings (3/4 cup each serving)

Nutrition Facts: Calories: 160 | Carbs: 18g | Protein: 4g | Fat: 8g | Sodium: 63mg

Ingredients:

- Four cups of fresh florets of broccoli
- One medium-sized apple
- Half a cup each of
  - Sweetened cranberries (dried)
  - Red onion
- A quarter cup each of
  - Walnuts
  - Fresh parsley
  - Mayonnaise
- Two tbsps. each of
  - Apple cider vinegar
  - Honey
- A three-fourth cup of plain Greek yogurt (low-fat)

Method:

1. Prepare the broccoli florets by cutting into bite-sized chunks. Trim them properly. Take the apple and cut into small pieces as well but in the unpeeled state. Prepare the parsley by chopping them coarsely.

2. Now, take a large-sized bowl and add the mayonnaise, yogurt, vinegar, honey, and parsley. Whisk them together.

3. Take the remaining ingredients and add them too. Make sure they are evenly coated with the yogurt mixture. Once prepared, keep the salad in the refrigerator because it is best served when chilled. It allows the flavors to combine properly. Before serving, stir the salad.

Notes:

- *You can use your favorite type of apple.*

- *If you want, you can sprinkle some more parsley on top just before serving.*

Pineapple Frangelico Sorbet

Total Prep & Cooking Time: 2 hours 10 minutes

Yields: 4 servings

Nutrition Facts: Calories: 119 | Carbs: 28g | Protein: 1g | Fat: 0.2g | Sodium: 2.4mg

Ingredients:

- Two tsps. of Stevia
- One tbsp. of Frangelico (keep two tsps. extra)
- Half a cup of unsweetened pineapple juice
- Two cups of pineapple (fresh)

Method:

1. Take all the ingredients in the container of the blender and process them until you get a smooth mixture.

2. Then, take this mixture and divide it into ice cubes. Keep it in the refrigerator and allow it to freeze.

3. When you find that the mixture has frozen, take them out and blend them in the food processor again. This process will give you a fluffy texture.

4. Before you serve, refreeze the sorbet.

Egg Muffins

Total Prep & Cooking Time: 45 minutes

Yields: 8 servings

Nutrition Facts: Calories: 154 | Carbs: 3g | Protein: 12g | Fat: 10g | Sodium: 155mg

Ingredients:

- Half an lb. of ground pork
- Half a tsp. of herb seasoning blend of your choice
- A quarter tsp. of salt
- Eight eggs (large-sized)
- A quarter tsp. each of
  o Onion powder
  o Garlic powder
  o Poultry seasoning
- One cup each of
  o Onion
  o Bell peppers (A mixture of orange, yellow, and red)

Method:

1. Set the oven temperature to 350 degrees F and use cooking spray to coat a muffin tin of regular size.

2. Prepare the onions and bell peppers by dicing them finely.

3. Take a bowl and in it, combine the following ingredients – garlic powder, poultry seasoning, pork, onion powder, and herb seasoning blend. Form the sausage by combining all of this properly.

4. Now cook the sausage in a non-stick skillet. Once it has been appropriately cooked, drain the sausage.

5. Use salt and milk substitute/milk to beat the eggs in a bowl. In it, add the veggies and the sausage mix.

6. Take the prepared muffin tin and pour the egg mixture into it. You have to leave enough space for the muffins so that they can rise. Bake them for about 20-22 minutes.

Notes: *If there are extra muffins, then you can have them as a quick breakfast the next day, and you simply have to reheat them for about 40 seconds.*

Linguine With Broccoli, Chickpeas, and Ricotta

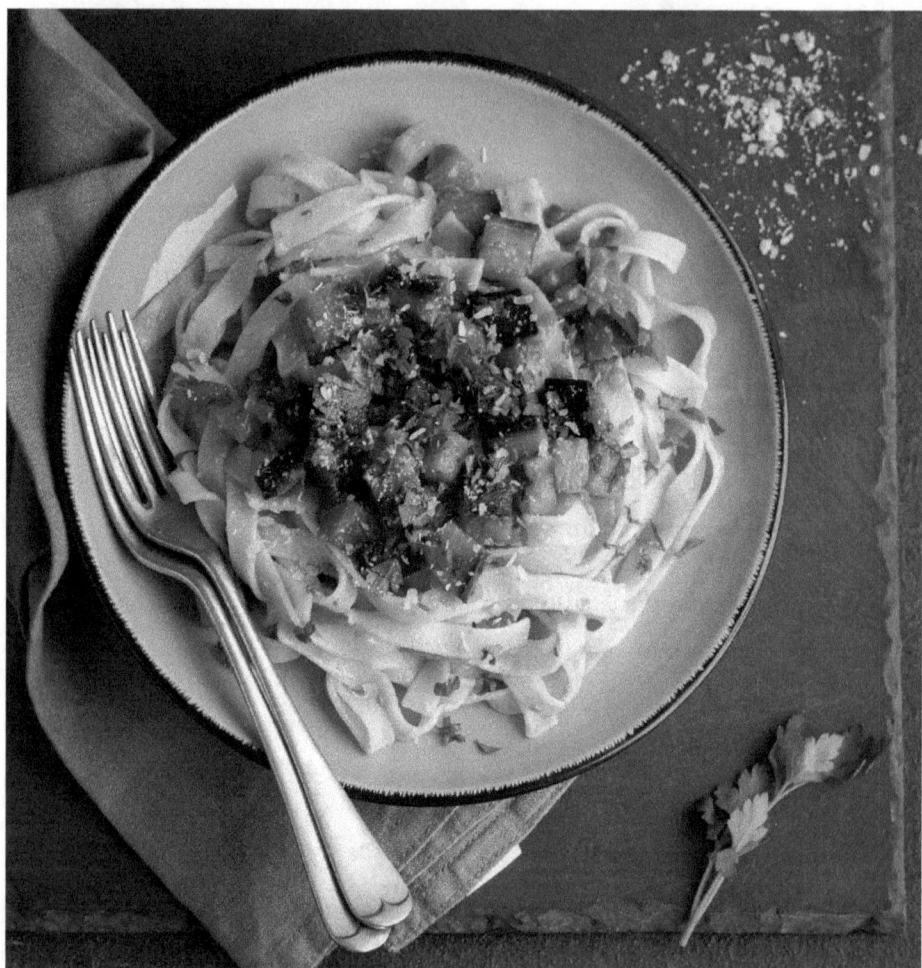

Total Prep & Cooking Time: 1 hour 5 minutes

Yields: 4 servings

Nutrition Facts: Calories: 404 | Carbs: 49.8g | Protein: 13.2g | Fat: 17.5g | Sodium: 180.4mg

Ingredients:

- Eight ounces of ricotta cheese that have been kept at room temperature
- A bunch of Tuscan kale (chopped into bite-sized chunks and stemmed)
- One-third cup of extra-virgin olive oil
- A pinch of black pepper
- Two cloves of garlic (sliced thinly)
- Fourteen ounces of chickpeas (rinsed after draining)
- Twelve ounces of spaghetti or linguine pasta
- A pinch of kosher salt
- One lemon
- Half a teaspoon of red pepper flakes
- Two tablespoons of unsalted butter
- To taste – Flaky sea salt

Method:

1. Take a large pot and add water to it. Add salt and bring the water to a boil. Cook the pasta by following the directions mentioned on the package. They must be perfectly al dente. Once the pasta is done, you have to drain it but, at the same time, reserve half a cup of the cooking water.

2. Heat the broiler and adjust the rack. Toss the following ingredients together in a bowl – garlic, chickpeas, broccoli, one-third cup of oil,

and red pepper flakes. Everything should become evenly coated. Use pepper and salt to season the mixture.

3. Take a sheet pan and spread the mixture out on it evenly.

4. Take the kale and add it to the previous bowl you used. Toss it again along with the remaining oil, if any. If you need it, then you can drizzle some more oil on top. Spread the kale in a second sheet pan in an even layer.

5. You have to take one sheet at a time while working. Broil the chickpeas and broccoli and halfway through the process, toss them. The broccoli should become charred and tender, and the chickpeas should be toasty. It will take about seven minutes. Then, broil the kale too for about five minutes, and they should become crispy.

6. Take the lemon, zest it, and then cut it into two halves. Take one half and form four wedges out of it. The juice of the lemon will have to be squeezed out on the roasted veggies and then use pepper and salt to season.

7. Place the pasta back in the pot. Take the pasta water you had earlier reserved and add it to the pasta and the lemon zest, butter, and ricotta. Keep tossing so that everything is well incorporated. Now, add the roasted veggies too. If you need, add some more pasta water while tossing.

8. Now, your linguine is done, and you have to divide it among four bowls—season with pepper and flaky sea salt. Squeeze a few drops of lemon on top and serve. If you want, drizzle some more oil before serving.

Ground Beef Soup
Total Prep & Cooking Time: 35 minutes

Yields: 6 servings

Nutrition Facts: Calories: 222 | Carbs: 19g | Protein: 20g | Fat: 8g | Sodium: 170mg

Ingredients:

- Half a cup of onion
- One tbsp. of sour cream
- Three cups of mixed vegetables (frozen, peas, green beans, corn, and carrots)
- One-third cup of uncooked white rice
- Two cups of water
- One cup of beef broth (reduced-sodium variety)
- One tsp. of browning sauce and seasoning of your choice
- Two tsps. of lemon pepper seasoning of your choice
- One lb. of ground beef (lean)

Method:

1. Prepare the onion by chopping them thoroughly. Then, take a large-sized saucepan and, in it, brown the onion and ground beef together. Drain the juices and excess fat.

2. Add the browning sauce and seasonings. Then, add the mixed veggies, rice, water, and beef broth and mix everything together.

3. Bring the mixture to a boil after placing it on high flame. Once the mixture starts boiling, reduce the flame to medium-low and cover the saucepan. Allow it to simmer and cook it for half an hour.

4. Once done, remove the pan from the flame and add the sour cream. Stir it in and serve.

Apple Oatmeal Crisp

Total Prep & Cooking Time: 40 minutes

Yields: 8 servings

Nutrition Facts: Calories: 297 | Carbs: 42g | Protein: 3g | Fat: 13g | Sodium: 95mg

Ingredients:

- A three-quarter cup of brown sugar
- Half a cup of butter
- One tsp. of cinnamon
- Half a cup of all-purpose flour
- Five apples (if possible, then Granny Smith ones)
- One cup of whole oatmeal

Method:

1. Set the temperature of the oven to 350 degrees F and preheat. Peel the apples, core them, and then cut them into slices.

2. Take a bowl and then mix the following ingredients in it together – brown sugar, oatmeal, cinnamon, and flour.

3. Use a pastry cutter to cut the butter into the oatmeal and make sure they are well blended.

4. Take a baking pan of 9 by 9 inches in size and place the sliced apples in it.

5. Take the oatmeal mixture and sprinkle it on top of the apples.

6. Bake the mixture for about thirty to thirty-five minutes.

Chapter 2: Weekend Recipes for Renal Diet

Hawaiian Chicken Salad Sandwich
Total Prep & Cooking Time: 10 minutes + chilling

Yields: 4 servings

Nutrition Facts: Calories: 349 | Carbs: 24g | Protein: 22g | Fat: 17g | Sodium: 398mg

Ingredients:

- One cup of pineapple tidbits
- Two cups of cooked chicken
- One-third cup of carrots
- Half a cup each of
  - Green bell pepper
  - Mayonnaise (low-fat)
- Four units of flatbread
- Half a tsp. of black pepper

Method:

1. Take the cooked chicken and chop it into bite-sized pieces.

2. Prepare the pineapple by draining it and then shred the carrots and chop the bell pepper.

3. Take all the ingredients in a medium-sized bowl and mix them well.

4. Refrigerate the mixture until it is thoroughly chilled.

5. Before serving, spread the chicken on the flatbread's open surface, or if you prefer it wrapped, you can use a tortilla too.

Apple Puffs

Total Prep & Cooking Time: 1 hour 20 minutes

Yields: 12 servings

Nutrition Facts: Calories: 156 | Carbs: 22g | Protein: 1.5g | Fat: 7.3g | Sodium: 176mg

Ingredients:

- Eight ounces of puff dough sheets
- One can (21 oz.) of apple pie filling
- Half a tsp. of rum extract
- One tsp. each of
  - Powdered sugar
  - Baking soda
  - Ground cinnamon

Method:

1. First, you have to thaw the puff dough sheets at room temperature, and it will take you approximately 1 hour.

2. Set the temperature of the oven to 400 degrees F and preheat.

3. Take a bowl, and in it, add the apple pie filling. If you have already sliced the apples, then you can form thirds from them now. Mix the rum extract and cinnamon with the apples.

4. Once the dough has been completely thawed, take one of the sheets and cut nine equal squares from it. Take the other sheet, and you will need only one-third of it to cut another three such squares.

5. Now, take the muffin tin and place the squares in each of the tins. In each of these squares, spoon some of the apple mixture.

6. Bake the preparation in the preheated oven for fifteen minutes, and they should become golden brown in color.

7. Once done, remove the puffs from the muffin tins and before serving, sprinkle some powdered sugar on top of each apple puff. Serve them warm.

Creamy Orzo and Vegetables

Total Prep & Cooking Time: 30 minutes

Yields: 6 servings

Nutrition Facts: Calories: 176 | Carbs: 25g | Protein: 10g | Fat: 4g | Sodium: 193mg

Ingredients:

- Half a cup of frozen green peas
- One tsp. of curry powder
- One carrot (medium-sized)
- One zucchini (small-sized)
- One onion (small-sized)
- One clove of garlic
- Three cups of chicken broth (low-sodium variety)
- Two tbsps. each of
  - Olive oil
  - Fresh parsley
- A quarter tsp. of black pepper
- A quarter cup of Parmesan cheese (freshly grated)
- One cup of cooked orzo pasta
- A quarter tsp. of salt

Method:

1. Start by preparing the veggies. Chop the zucchini and onion. Chop the garlic finely. Then, take the carrots and shred them.

2. Place a large-sized skillet on the oven over medium flame. Heat olive oil in the skillet. Sauté the following ingredients in it for about five minutes – carrots, zucchini, onion, and garlic.

3. After that, add the curry powder to the mixture. Season with salt and then add the chicken broth. Bring the mixture to a boil.

4. Now, add the cooked orzo pasta and keep stirring until the mixture starts boiling. Cover the skillet and allow the mixture to simmer. Keep stirring from time to time and cook the pasta for another 10 minutes. By this time, the pasta will become al dente, and the liquid will be absorbed.

5. Add the chopped parsley, cheese, and the frozen peas into the pasta. Keep heating until the vegetables are sufficiently hot, and if you want to enhance the creaminess, then you can add some more broth—season with pepper.

Minestrone Soup

Total Prep & Cooking Time: 45 minutes

Yields: 4 servings

Nutrition Facts: Calories: 144 | Carbs: 21.9g | Protein: 5.9g | Fat: 4.3g |
Sodium: 55.1mg

Ingredients:

- Four cups of low-sodium chicken broth (low-fat)
- One carrot (large-sized)
- One and a half cups of dry macaroni (elbow-shaped)
- 14 oz. of tomatoes (diced, without any salt content)
- Two stalks of celery
- Two garlic cloves
- Half a cup of zucchini (freshly chopped)
- One teaspoon each of
  - Dried basil
  - Dried oregano
  - Freshly ground black pepper
- Half an onion (large-sized)
- One can of green snap beans (without any salt content)
- Two tbsps. of olive oil

Method:

1. Prepare the veggies by dicing zucchini, garlic, and onion. Then, take the carrots and shred them. Either use fresh green beans or canned ones, but you have to cut them into pieces of half an inch size.

2. Take a Dutch oven or a large pot and place it on medium flame—heat olive oil in the pot. Add the diced onions in the pot as well and then cook them for a couple of minutes until they become translucent.

3. Add zucchini, carrot, celery, and garlic, and if you are using fresh green beans, then add them too. Cook the vegetables for about five minutes and they will become tender.

4. Add black pepper, oregano, basil, and if you are using canned beans, then add them now.

5. Add the chicken broth and the diced tomatoes and keep stirring.

6. Bring the mixture to a boil and once it starts boiling, allow the mixture to simmer for about ten minutes.

7. Add the pasta and cook them for an additional ten minutes by following the directions mentioned on the package.

8. Before serving, garnish the pasta with fresh basil on top. Serve into bowls and enjoy!

Frosted Grapes

Total Prep & Cooking Time: 1 hour 5 minutes

Yields: 10 servings (serving size – half a cup)

Nutrition Facts: Calories: 88 | Carbs: 21g | Protein: 1g | Fat: 0g | Sodium: 41mg

Ingredients:

- Three oz. of flavored gelatin
- Five cups of seedless grapes

Method:

1. De-steam the seedless grapes after you have washed them. After that, let them be but make sure they are slightly damp.

2. In a large-sized bowl, add the dry gelatin mix. Remember that you shouldn't be pouring in water.

3. Add these damp grapes into the bowl, and in order to coat them uniformly, toss them well.

4. Now, take a baking sheet, and place these grapes on the sheet in an even layer.

5. Freeze them for 1 hour and then serve chilled.

Notes: *The flavor of the gelatin you use can be adjusted as per your choice. If you want to decrease the carbs, then use gelatin that is sugar-free.*

Yogurt and Fruit Salad

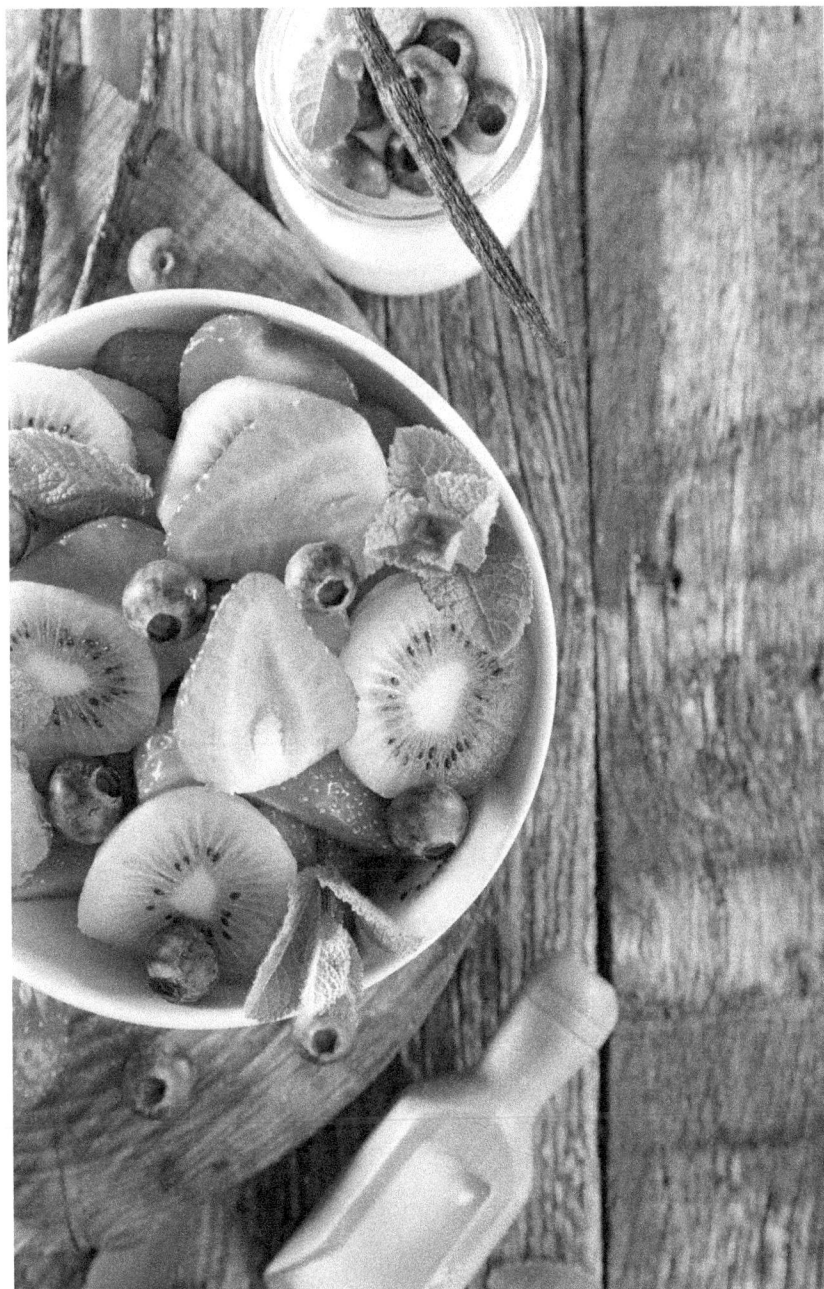

Total Prep & Cooking Time: 2 hours 20 minutes

Yields: 4 servings

Nutrition Facts: Calories: 99 | Carbs: 22g | Protein: 2.6g | Fat: 0.7g | Sodium: 12mg

Ingredients:

- One-third cup of dried cranberries
- Half a cup of pineapple chunks (fresh)
- Six strawberries (large-sized)
- Six ounces of Greek yogurt (strawberry flavored)
- Four ounces of mandarin oranges (drained, light syrup)
- Ten green grapes
- One apple (with skin, medium-sized)

Method:

1. Wash the strawberries, grapes, and apples. After that, pat them dry.

2. Slice the apples and chop them into bite-sized chunks.

3. Then, take the strawberries and slice them as well.

4. Mix the following ingredients together – yogurt, dried cranberries, pineapple, Mandarin oranges, grapes, and apples.

5. Keep the mixture covered and put it in the refrigerator for two hours.

6. Before serving, garnish the preparation with sliced strawberries.

Beet and Apple Juice Blend

Total Prep & Cooking Time: 5 minutes

Yields: 2 servings

Nutrition Facts: Calories: 53 | Carbs: 13g | Protein: 1g | Fat: 0g | Sodium: 66mg

Ingredients:

- A quarter cup of parsley
- Half a beet (medium-sized)
- Half an apple (medium-sized)
- One carrot (fresh, medium-sized)
- One stalk of celery

Method:

1. Process the following ingredients together in a juicer – parsley, celery, carrot, beet, and apple.

2. Take the mixture and pour it into two small glasses. You can either keep the juice in the refrigerator to chill or have it right away.

Notes: *Even though juices are healthy, for kidney patients, you have to be careful so that you don't increase your potassium intake too much.*

Baked Turkey Spring Rolls
Total Prep & Cooking Time: 1 hour 30 minutes

Yields: 8 servings (per serving – 2 spring rolls)

Nutrition Facts: Calories: 197 | Carbs: 9.6g | Protein: 23.3g | Fat: 7.3g | Sodium: 82.2mg

Ingredients:

- 2.5 cups of coleslaw mix
- Two tsps. of freshly ground black pepper
- Twenty ounces of turkey breast (ground)
- Two tbsps. each of
  - Vegetable oil
  - Minced cilantro
- One tbsp. each of
  - Sesame oil
  - Balsamic vinegar
- Two tsps. of freshly ground black pepper
- Sixteen pastry wrappers (frozen spring roll wraps)
- Cooking spray

Method:

1. Set the temperature of the oven to 400 degrees F and preheat.

2. Take the spring roll wrappers out from the freezer so that they can stay under room temperature. Thawing should be done at least half an hour before preparation.

3. Now, take a bowl, and in it, mix the following ingredients with the raw turkey – minced cilantro, sesame oil, and balsamic vinegar.

4. Take a large-sized skillet, and in it, pour two tbsps. of vegetable oil. Put the skillet on medium-high flame and preheat. Add the ground turkey

into the skillet and crumble it by stirring. To cook the turkey properly, you have to keep sautéing the mixture.

5. Then, you have to add the mixture of coleslaw to the turkey and keep cooking for another five minutes. Season with freshly ground black pepper – two tsps. should be enough. Mix everything properly.

6. Once done, remove the skillet from the flame. Use a strainer to drain any remaining liquid.

7. Take one spring roll wrapper and near one corner of it – add the filling diagonally. You can take three tbsps. of filling for one roll. There should be adequate space left on both sides. Fold one side towards the inside and do the same with the other side. Roll them and make sure the sights have been tucked in properly. Use water to moisten one of the sides of the wrapper because this helps to seal properly.

8. Take the remaining wrappers and follow the same steps with them.

9. Use non-stick cooking spray to coat the baking pan's base and then place the spring rolls in it. Place the pan in the oven, and it should be complete in half an hour when given at 400 degrees F.

10. You can also serve the rolls with a sweet chili sauce, but this has not been included in the nutrition facts.

Crab-Stuffed Celery Logs

Total Prep & Cooking Time: 10 minutes

Yields: 4 servings

Nutrition Facts: Calories: 34 | Carbs: 2g | Protein: 2g | Fat: 2g | Sodium: 94mg

Ingredients:

- Two tsps. of mayonnaise
- One tbsp. of red onion
- A quarter cup of crab meat
- Four ribs or celery (approx. eight inches in size)
- A quarter tsp. of paprika
- Half a tsp. of lemon juice

Method:

1. Take the celery ribs and trim the ends. Prepare the crab meat by draining it and then use two forks to flake the meat. Chop the onion and mince it thoroughly.

2. Take a small-sized bowl and in it, add the lemon juice, mayonnaise, onion, and crab meat and combine them properly.

3. Take a whole tablespoon full of the mixture and fill the celery rib with it.

4. Each rib of celery has to be cut into three equal pieces.

5. Sprinkle some paprika on top of each of these celery logs.

Couscous Salad

Total Prep & Cooking Time: 50 minutes

Yields: 4 servings (half a cup per serving)

Nutrition Facts: Calories: 151 | Carbs: 28.7g | Protein: 4.9g | Fat: 2.5g | Sodium: 14.3mg

Ingredients:

- One teaspoon each of
  - Dried oregano
  - Allspice
- Two lemons (juiced)
- One tbsp. each of
  - Olive oil
  - Minced garlic
- Half a cup each of
  - Red bell pepper (chopped)
  - Yellow bell pepper (chopped)
  - Carrots (chopped)
  - Frozen corn
- One cup each of
  - Dry couscous
  - Whole sugar snap peas
- Three peeled cucumbers (large-sized)

Method:

1. Follow the package instructions to prepare the couscous. After that, allow it to chill.

2. Take a large bowl and mix the following ingredients: cucumbers, couscous, snow peas, carrots, corn, yellow pepper, and red pepper.

3. Take another bowl of small size and, in it, whisk the following ingredients together – dried oregano, allspice, lemon juice, olive oil, and minced garlic.

4. Combine everything and serve it chilled.

Chapter 3: One-Week Meal Plan

Day 1

Breakfast – Pumpkin Pancakes

Lunch – Ground Beef Soup

Snacks – Frosted Grapes

Dinner – Pasta Salad

Day 2

Breakfast – Yogurt and Fruit Salad

Lunch – Broccoli and Apple Salad

Snacks – Apple Puffs

Dinner – Baked Turkey Spring Rolls

Day 3

Breakfast – Egg Muffins

Lunch – Minestrone Soup

Snacks – Crab-Stuffed Celery Logs

Dinner – Hawaiian Chicken Salad Sandwich

Day 4

Breakfast – Yogurt and Fruit Salad

Lunch – Pasta Salad

Snacks – Apple Puffs

Dinner – Linguine with Broccoli, Chickpeas, and Ricotta

Day 5

Breakfast – Beet and Apple Juice Blend

Lunch – Ground Beef Soup

Snacks – Frosted Grapes

Dinner – Baked Turkey Spring Rolls

Day 6

Breakfast – Pumpkin Pancakes

Lunch – Creamy Orzo and Vegetables

Snacks – Pineapple Frangelico Sorbet

Dinner – Couscous Salad

Day 7

Breakfast – Egg Muffins

Lunch – Broccoli and Apple Salad

Snacks – Pineapple Frangelico Sorbet

Dinner – Ground Beef Soup

Chapter 4: Avoiding Dialysis and Taking the Right Supplements

Even though getting diagnosed with chronic kidney disease (CKD) might appear scary, you can take certain steps to prolong your kidney function and delay the onset of dialysis if you catch the disease in its early stages. Some of the main causes of CKD in Americans are high blood pressure and diabetes. In order to prolong kidney function, these diseases should be controlled.

Steps to Avoid Dialysis and Prolong Kidney Function

There are steps an individual could take to prolong kidney function regardless of how the individual developed CKD.

- **Following a renal diet** – The main aim of a pre-dialysis diet is to maintain optimum nutrition. A renal diet is one that has a low content of protein, phosphorus, and sodium and emphasizes the importance of limiting the intake of fluids and consuming high-quality protein. It's essential to consult your dietician for individualized nutrition counseling. Several doctors believe that the progression of kidney diseases can be slowed down by following a renal diet.

- **Reduce the intake of salt** – Consuming an excess amount of salt with your foods is linked with high blood pressure.

- **Exercise regularly** – Exercises like running, walking, and swimming can help maintain a healthy weight, manage diabetes and high blood pressure, and decrease stress.

- **Reduce stress** – Decreasing stress and anxiety can lower your blood pressure, which in turn can be beneficial for your kidneys.

- **Don't smoke** – Smoking decreases the flow of blood to your kidneys. It decreases kidney function in both people with or without diseases.

- **Limit alcohol intake** – Alcohol consumption can increase your blood pressure. The excess calories can also make you gain weight.

- **Drink enough water** – Your kidneys can be damaged by dehydration, decreasing blood flow to the kidneys. However, follow your nutritionist's guidelines regarding fluid intake because regular fluid intake can also increase the build-up of fluid in your body, which can become dangerous for patients in the later stages of CKD.

- **Control your blood pressure** – High blood pressure can increase your risk of kidney failure and heart diseases.

- **Control your blood sugar** – The risk of kidney failure and heart diseases are increased due to diabetes.

- **Maintain a healthy weight** – The risk of kidney-related conditions like high blood pressure and diabetes can be increased because of obesity.

Even though CKD cannot be reversed, appropriate treatment can slow down its progression. See your doctor regularly to monitor your kidney function and slow the progression of kidney failure.

The dietary requirements of people who are suffering from any sort of kidney problems are not always the same. Someone might need extra calories and proteins, whereas others might need fewer amounts of such nutrients. Thus, a professional healthcare provider is the best person who can assist and guide you for choosing the perfect supplements necessary for your kidney disease. Special supplements meant for keeping the kidney safe are available in various sizes, shapes, flavors, and forms. It is always necessary to consult a healthcare practitioner before consuming any nutritional supplement related to the kidney.

Individuals who are suffering from chronic kidney disease (CKD) require certain water-soluble vitamins in higher quantities. Here you will get to know about some of the supplements that are meant for dealing with kidney problems.

- **Vitamin B1 or Thiamin -** It looks after the proper functioning of the nervous system. Thiamin also helps the cells in producing the required amount of energy from carbohydrates. People with chronic kidney disease are recommended to intake 1.5mg of this water-soluble vitamin supplement per day.

- **Vitamin B2 or Riboflavin -** Vitamin B2 supports healthy skin as well as normal vision. People who are fighting against CKD and are also following a special low-protein diet might consume 1.8mg of Riboflavin supplement each day. Those of you who have a low appetite and are pursuing dialysis might take 1.1 to 1.3mg of vitamin B2 supplements per day.

- **Vitamin B6 -** This effective water-soluble vitamin helps produce proteins that are further used for making cells. Patients of CKD who are under dialysis treatment might consume 10mg of this supplement each day. Those who are non-dialysis patients are recommended to intake 5mg vitamin B6 supplements every day.

- **NAC -** NAC or N-acetylcysteine is an essential amino acid that generally targets the oxygen radicals. Various findings and researches suggest that NAC supplementation is beneficial for hemodialysis patients. NAC supplement decreases oxidative stress as well as improves results of uremic anemia, which is a problem of CKD.

- **ALA -** The antioxidant Alpha lipoic acid might prove helpful in treating certain complications of kidney disease. Supplementation of ALA enhances the action of a few antioxidant enzymes. Such enzymes protect against oxidative disorders and stress.

- **Vitamin B12 -** Vitamin B12 maintains the nerve cells and, in association with folate, produces red blood cells. Both dialysis and non-dialysis CKD patients are recommended to intake 2-3 mg of this supplement per day. Its deficiency can result in permanent nerve damage.

Supplements for kidney problems are better to consume only if it is approved or prescribed by your doctor.

PART II

Chapter 1: Introduction to the Low FODMAP diet

Do you suffer from abdominal cramping and discomfort? If you spend your days feeling constipated, bloated, and feel the uncontrollable urge to use the bathroom? If so, you may suffer from IBS.

With so many diets on the market, it can be hard to decide which one is best for you! In the following chapters, you will be learning everything you need to know about the FODMAP diet and how it can benefit your life.

Unfortunately, there are several theories behind why individuals suffer from IBS. For many, there is 70% of women who suffer from IBS due to their hormones triggering the symptoms. As for others, the reasons could be anything from a sensitive colon, an immune response to stressors, sensitive brain activity in detecting gut contractions, or even a neurotransmitter serotonin being produced in the gut. While the doctors are unable to pinpoint an exact reason for IBS, the good news is that they are certain that IBS will not cause other gastrointestinal diseases and it is not cancer!

The right question to ask in this moment, is what can I do about it? We are here to tell you that the low FODMAP diet is the way to go. In the chapters to follow, you will learn everything from what the diet is, who the diet is for, what FODMAP even stands for, and why this diet will work for you. We cover the benefits of the diet and include an easy start guide so you can get rid of that discomfort and bloat as soon as possible!

To start, it is important to understand what the FODMAP diet is, and why it is something you need to start. However, before we start, here are some tips for the beginners who are just starting or considering the low FODMAP diet.

Getting Started

Before we begin, it is important to get a diagnosis from your family doctor. Many people self-diagnose themselves with IBS and place themselves on the low FODMAP diet. This is something we do not recommend. If you have symptoms such as pain and bloating, you should see a professional to rule out any possible life-threatening diseases.

What is IBS?

As mentioned, be sure to see a professional to attain an official prognosis of IBS. If you suspect you do have Irritable Bowel Syndrome, realize that you are not alone. In fact, around 15% of the population in the United States suffer from IBS symptoms. While the symptoms do vary from person to person, the typical symptoms are as follow:

- Bloating
- Constipation
- Diarrhea
- Lower Abdominal Pain
- Lower Abdominal Discomfort

If you suffer from any of these, it is important to consult with your doctor the specific symptoms you have. This will be vital as there are three different types of irritable bowel syndrome. These include:

- IBS with Constipation
  - Typically, IBS with constipation has symptoms including bloating, abnormally delayed bowel movements, stomach pains, and loose or lumpy stool.
- IBS with Diarrhea
  - Typically comes with symptoms including stomach pain, urgent need to use the bathroom, loose and watery stool
- IBS with alternating Diarrhea and Constipation

Due to the fact that there are several types of IBS, this makes it hard to determine a single drug treatment to help with the symptoms. As we mentioned earlier, you need to consult with a professional. Once you have done this and ruled out any other illnesses, it is time to take a look at your diet.

Who is the diet for?

Typically, the low FODMAP diet is meant for individuals suffering from IBS. The diet itself was created as one of the first food-based treatments to help relieve IBS symptoms. The good news is that up to 75% of patients who had IBS experienced symptom relief when they followed the low FODMAP diet. However, the diet is also helpful if you have any of the following:

- Digestive Disorder
  - Gastroesophageal Reflux Disease (GERD)
  - Crohn's Disease
  - Celiac Disease

- Vegan Gut
- Bloating

Once you have determined that the low FODMAP diet could help your symptoms, it is now time to learn what FODMAP even stands for! This is going to be vital information to carry with you through your diet so you understand what you are eating and why your body is reacting the way it does!

We understand that there are many different types of diets out there. Some of you may be wondering, can I follow my current diet and still follow the low FODMAP diet? The answer varies depending on which you follow, and we will try to answer in a simple manner:

- Vegetarian/ Vegan
  - Yes, this diet is more than possible to follow if you are vegan or vegetarian. With a few tweaks, you can find friendly options and still stick to your regular diet!
- Low-Salt
  - If you follow a low-salt diet, this diet is doable for you. However, it will be vital that you learn how to read and follow food labels. Luckily for you, this is information also included in this book!
- Gluten-Free
  - As you will be learning, the FODMAP diet does exclude wheat, which contains gluten. If you are gluten-free, this diet is easy to follow as you most likely will not be able to have it anyway!

- Kosher
  - If you have to eat kosher, you can still follow this diet. It will be up to you to find certain kosher foods, but after the elimination diet, you will be able to find the foods and still stick to your original diet.

History of the low FODMAP diet

Originally, the low FODMAP diet was developed by a team of scientists at the Monash University located in Australia. The original research was meant to investigate if the diet would be able to control IBS symptoms with food alone. The university established a food analysis program to study FODMAPs in both Australian as well as international foods.

In 2005, the first FODMAP ideas would be published as part of a research paper. In the paper, the hypothesis was that by reducing dietary intake of certain foods that were deemed indigestible, this could help reduce symptoms stimulated in an individual's gut's nervous system.

Over many years, research has shown that certain short-chain carbohydrates such as lactose, sorbitol, and fructose was the cause behind gastrointestinal discomfort. Once the basis of digestion was studied, the low FODMAP diet was created to help with these symptoms.

What does FODMAP stand for?

FODMAPs are typically found in foods that we consume every day. They are in onions, rye, barley, wheat, garlic, milk, fruits, vegetables, and more! As you can tell from this very small list (don't worry, we will cover more in the chapters to follow), they are in some of our more common foods!

This is why it is so easy to feel bloated for some people, without understanding what is causing it! However, before we dive into how this diet works, you will need to understand the acronym FODMAP.

F-Fermentable

O- Oligosaccharies (short chain carbohydrates)

D- Disaccharides (lactose)

M- Monosaccharides (fructose)

A- and

P- Polyols (Sorbitol, xylitol, maltitol, and mannitol)

The reason you may be suffering from IBS or other digestive issues is due to the fact that most FODMAPs have a hard time absorbing into your small intestine. As a result, these FODMAPs are fermented by the bacteria in your small and large intestine in which results in bloating and irregular bowel movements.

While the FODMAPs cause the digestive discomfort, it is important to understand that it is not the cause of the intestinal inflammation itself. In fact, the FODMAPs produce alterations of intestinal flora that help you maintain a healthy colon. This does not change that the symptoms are still uncomfortable.

What may be causing your IBS symptoms could be a fructose malabsorption or a lactose intolerance. As you will be learning in later chapters, as you begin the low FODMAP diet, there will be an elimination phase where you learn what exactly is causing your symptoms and discomfort.

The source of the FODMAP will vary depending on different dietary groups. In more common circumstances they are compromised as the following:

- Oligosaccharies: Fructans and Galacto-oligosaccharies
- Disaccharies- Lactose
- Monosaccharies- Fructose
- Polyols- Xylitol, Mannitol, Sorbitol

Sources of Fructans

In later chapters, we will be going more in-depth on the foods you can and cannot eat. To cover the basics, you should understand where these specific irritants come from. To start, we will go over the source of fructans. These can be found in very popular ingredients including; rye, garlic, onion, wheat, beetroot, Brussel sprouts, and certain prebiotics.

Sources of Galactans

As for galactans, these are primarily found in beans and pulses. It can also be found in certain tofu and tempeh, but this does not mean that vegans and vegetarians cannot follow the low FODMAP diet. It simply means that you will need to find other sources of proteins if you want to follow a plant-based diet. We will be going over this more in the chapters to follow.

Sources of Polyols

Polyols are typically found in stone fruits. These include avocados, apples, blackberries, watermelon, and more. They are also found naturally in certain vegetables and bulk sweeteners.

While this diet may seem to be lacking many of your favorite foods, don't you worry! Due to the wide variety of IBS symptoms, it is unclear which foods trigger certain individuals. This is why the elimination trial will be important before you start the diet. Please remember that everyone is different. While some people see immediate results when they begin the diet, for others, it will take some time.

Effectiveness and Risks of the low FODMAP diet

It is important to understand that the low FODMAP diet is meant for short-term symptom relief. However, long-term diet can have a negative effect on your body. Unfortunately, it can be detrimental to your guy metabolome and microbiota. It is to be taken very seriously that this diet is meant for short periods of time and only under the advice of a professional.

Please understand that if you choose to follow the low FODMAP diet without any medical advice, it is possible the diet could lead to some serious health risks. Some of these risks are as followed:

- Nutritional Deficiencies

- Increased Risk of Cancer
- Death

When you start the low FODMAP diet, it is possible the diet itself could mask any serious disease that present themselves of digestive symptoms. These could include celiac disease, colon cancer, or inflammatory bowel disease. This is why it is so crucial to seek professional help before starting the diet on your own.

Now that you have learned the basics of the low FODMAP diet, it is time to learn all about the benefits that come with the diet change. Obviously, the main change will be to help lower any digestive troubles you may behaving. By removing the potential triggers in which are causing your digestive issues, this will help pinpoint which food intolerances you have.

While this diet may seem to take a lot of time and effort, think of the time you are wasting by being in discomfort all of the time and using the bathroom! With a few minor adjustments and tests, you will be able to find the source of your problem and hopefully never feel this way again! Now, onto learn all of the other incredible benefits the low FODMAP diet can bring to you!

Chapter 2: Benefits of the Low FODMAP diet

According to research, the low FODMAP diet is effective for around 75% of patients who suffer from IBS. In most cases, the patients are able reduce any major symptoms they are experiencing and in hand, improve their quality of life.

In the same research, scientist found evidence that the diet can also be beneficial for people who suffer from other functional gastrointestinal disorders such as Chron's disease, ulcerative colitis, and inflammatory bowel disease. All you need to do to benefit from this diet is to figure out what is causing the digestive disturbances and symptoms. Below, you will find some of the other benefits the low FODMAP diet has to offer:

A. IBS Symptom Reduction

By following the low FODMAP diet, individuals can reduce most symptoms involved with IBS including stomach pain, bloating, and gas. It is important to follow the diet and remove any irritants as they ferment inside of your intestines. By selecting foods that don't trigger your symptoms, you can avoid them altogether!

B. Chron's Disease Reduced Discomfort
By following the low FODMAP diet, individuals were able to change the quality and number of prebiotics. By controlling the foods you consume and avoiding the ones that trigger your system, you could reduce the discomfort you feel from the trigger foods.

C. Increased Energy

Some individuals feel tired no matter how much they eat through the day. It is believed that a low FODMAP diet can help reduce fatigue. This could be due to the fact that the body is no longer wasting energy on digesting foods that don't agree with your system. This is especially true for sweeteners that you could be using on a daily basis. As you will be learning later, some of the best sweeteners can be found in fruit!

D. Reduced Constipation and Diarrhea

When you follow the low FODMAP diet, you will begin to eliminate foods that are causing your symptoms in the first place. When you do this, your body will find a balance, and you may find that your bloating will decrease, the gas will decrease, and your stools will return to normal. It is a win-win situation! All you will need to do is figure out your triggers (which we cover in the third chapter) and follow the diet!

On top of these incredible benefits, there is also beliefs that the low FODMAP diet can benefit psychological health. Often times, the disturbances of IBS can cause stress to certain individuals, eventually leading to anxiety and depression. When you remove the trigger causing the symptoms by diet, you will be able to improve the quality of your life.

As you will be learning in the chapters to follow, the low FODMAP diet includes an elimination diet in order to get started. As you introduce foods, you may find that you have a lactose or gluten intolerance. While this may seem like a huge change, there are some incredible benefits to changing your diet.

Benefits of a Grain Free Diet

As you will be learning later in the book, there are many types of grains that has been found to cause inflammation. Unfortunately, this is a very common culprit for the digestive disorders you may be experiencing. This is especially true if you are very sensitive to gluten. The good news is that if you are looking to lose weight on top of feeling better, cutting out these grains will be the best thing to ever happen to you. Reined grains are high in carbohydrates and calories; they offer little to no nutrition and contribute to discomfort in your stomach. Before you make the switch to going grain free, consider some of the amazing benefits as follow:

A. Digestion Benefits

Gluten is a type of protein that can be found in wheat products. If you do the elimination diet and find that you are gluten sensitive, cutting it out makes the most sense. When you cut it out of your diet, this can help relieve issues such as nausea, bloating, diarrhea and constipation.

B. Reduced Inflammation

When you experience acute inflammation, this normally means that your immune system is fighting off foreign invaders. Unfortunately, if you sustain these levels for a long period of time, this is what causes chronic disease. By cutting gluten out, you can reduce the amount of inflammation in your body.

C. Balanced Microbiome

By following a grain-free diet, you will be able to balance the microbiome in your gut. When you do this, it helps support the beneficial bacteria in your body, helping improve your digestion, boost your immunity, and helps keep blood sugar under control.

D. Weight Loss

As mentioned earlier, most grains offer little to no nutrition. When you cut these extra calories out of your diet, it will help you lose weight. Instead of grains, try eating nutrient-dense foods like vegetables or legumes. Of course, you will figure out exactly what you can eat on the low FODMAP diet after going through the elimination portion.

Another common irritant when individuals suffer from IBS and other digestive orders can be lactose! You may be thinking to yourself; I could never give up my yogurt or ice cream. The good news is that in the current market, some incredible alternative choices can fit in the low FODMAP diet. In case you need some further benefits to help convince you, here are just a few:

E. Healthier Digestion

You may not know, but around 70% of the population has a degrees of intolerance to lactose. When we first begin to wean off of our mother's milk, we begin to use lactase. Lactase is an enzyme that helps digest lactose found in milk. As we age, we begin to lose the ability to digest lactose and is one of the biggest known triggers for IBS. By taking dairy out of your diet, you save yourself the troubles all together!

F. Decreased Bloating

Bloating occurs when we have issues with digestion. Some dairy products can cause excessive gas in the intestines, which is what causes the bloating in the first place. Some bodies are unable to break down the carbohydrates and sugar fully which in turn, creates an imbalance of gut bacteria.

G. Clearer Skin

If you suffer from acne, dairy could be the culprit! According to studies posted in Clinics in Dermatology, it was found that dairy products such as milk contain growth hormones that stimulate acne. By following the low FODMAP diet and cutting dairy from your diet, you could naturally treat acne!

H. Reduce Risk of Cancer

A 2001 study at Harvard School of Public Health found that there was a connection between high calcium intake and increased risk of prostate cancer. It is thought that the hormones in the milk contain contaminants such as pesticides that have been linked to cancer cell growth. These contaminants are mostly found in dairy products, giving you another reason to cut them from your diet altogether!

I. Decreased Oxidative Stress

It is believed that a high milk intake is typically associated with higher mortality rates in both men and women. This may be due to the D-galatose found in milk which helps influence oxidative stress and inflammation in the body. Unfortunately, this undesirable effect caused by milk can cause chronic expose and damage health. On top of inflammation, it can also shorten life spans, cause neurodegeneration and also decrease one's immune system.

As you can tell, there are so many incredible benefits of switching over to the low FODMAP diet. Whether you are looking to get rid of bloating, lose some weight, or stop constipation and/or diarrhea, the low FODMAP diet has got you covered. It is all a matter of figuring out what your trigger is in the first place.

Obviously, we could go on and on about the incredible benefits of the diet, but then we would never get to the diet itself! Now that you are aware of just some of the benefits, it is time to get you started! In the chapter to follow, you will be learning how to get started on the low FODMAP diet. You will the steps to get started on the diet itself and how to diet whether you are vegan, vegetarian, diabetics, or doing this for a child who suffers from IBS. When you are ready, we can dive in!

Chapter 3: Starting the Low FODMAP diet

Now that you are aware of the low FODMAP diet and some of its benefits, it is time to learn how you can get started on the diet yourself! While a diet and lifestyle change can seem daunting, it will be important to believe in yourself and remember why you started it in the first place. In the chapter to follow, we will be providing you with all of the information you need. From diagnosis of IBS, to starting the diet, and even how to practice if you are vegan, vegetarian, or diabetic. This diet can be universal; it is all about finding what works best for you. First, it is time to understand the diagnosis of IBS.

Getting Diagnosed with IBS and FODMAP Tests

If you are in the process of being diagnosed with a chronic medical condition, this could be a challenging time for you. It is important that you understand the symptoms the doctors are looking for, and which medical tests you will be taking in order to be officially diagnosed with irritable bowel syndrome. IBS can be diagnosed with a combination of Rome IV criteria so the doctors will be able to rule out any other gastrointestinal disorders.

Rome IV is a set of criteria that doctors have found that most IBS patients have in common. This criteria is 98% accurate when the doctors are identifying their patients with IBS. These criteria are as followed:

1. Recurrent abdominal pain at least one day per week in the last three months are have the following:
   A. Related to defecation

B. A change in stool frequency

C. Change in form of stool

2. Criteria from above is fulfilled with symptoms for at least six months before official diagnosis

Other symptoms often associated with IBS include bloating, abdominal pain, and a change in bowel habit. Your doctor will take in the evidence and match with the Rome IV criteria and will move onto discussing any red flag symptoms that may be occurring.

Before being diagnosed with IBS, it will be important that your doctor rules out any other medical conditions that could be presented with the same symptoms; this is where the red flag symptoms come into play. These flags include:

- Inflammatory Markers
- Rectal Masses
- Abdominal Masses
- Anemia
- Nocturnal Symptoms such as waking up from sleep to defecate
- Family History of coeliac disease, inflammatory bowel disease, and ovarian cancer
- Rectal Bleeding
- Unintentional Weight Loss

On top of these symptoms, your doctor will also ask for several other symptoms in order to diagnose you with IBS. Firstly, the discomfort and pain in your abdomen will need to be related to altered bowel frequency as well as a change in your stool form. You will also need to have at least two of the following symptoms:

1. Feeling incomplete emptying when using the bathroom
2. Passage of mucus when using the bathroom
3. Straining, Urgency, and Altered Stool passage
4. Abdominal Bloating
5. Lethargy
6. Backaches
7. Bladder Symptoms
8. Nausea

Medical Tests for IBS

Once your doctor figures out your symptoms, rules out any other serious medical conditions and believes it is appropriate to run tests for IBS can you expect one of the following tests:

- Antibody testing for coeliac disease
- C-reactive protein
- Erythrocyte sedimentation rate
- Full blood count

While these tests are typical, it may be different if you present any of the red flag symptoms from above. If you do have a red flag symptom, there will be additional tests to rule out any more serious issues. These tests are as follow:

- Hydrogen Breath Test (meant for lactose intolerance)
- Fecal Occult Blood

- Fecal Ova and Parasite Test
- Thyroid Function Test
- Rigid/ Flexible Sigmoidoscopy
- Ultrasound

In the case that your doctor feels your symptoms may not be linked to IBS, they will most likely refer you to a gastroenterologist. This is a physician who is an expert in managing diseases found in the liver and gastrointestinal tract. However, this is worst case scenario. For now, we will focus on following the diet if you are diagnosed with IBS.

Breaking down FODMAPS

In general, FODMAPs naturally occur in popular foods such as vegetables, fruits, grains, cereals, dairy products, and legumes. Unfortunately for those who suffer from IBS, these FODMAPs are absorbed poorly in our small intestines and can affect our bowels as a symptom. FODMAPs are short-chain carbohydrates found in these foods, but this does not mean that the diet itself is sugar-free. When we consume FODMAPs, they are fermented by gut bacteria in the large intestine in which triggers the unpleasant GI symptoms that you may be experiencing. Before we move onto the elimination stage, it is important to understand just what this acronym means.

Fermentable

Fermenting is the process where our gut bacteria attempt so break down FODMAPs. As you are already aware, these FODMAPs are indigestible carbohydrates and in turn, produce gas.

Oligo-Saccharies

This group of the FODMAP are broken down into two subgroups including fructans and galactans. Fructans also known as fructo-oligosaccharies or FOS are most commonly found in foods such as dried fruit, barley rye, wheat, garlic, onion. Galactans or galacto-oligosaccharies or GOS are found in pulses, legumes, cashews, pistachios, and silken tofu. If you feel yourself panicking over remembering these foods, don't worry. In the chapter to follow, we will cover exactly what you can and cannot eat while on the low FODMAP diet.

Di-Saccharies

As mentioned in the chapter from before, lactose could be a potential trigger in your diet. These can be found in any product that comes from goat, sheep, or cow's milk. Lactose itself contains two sugars united that require an enzyme known as lactase before our bodies are even able to absorb it. When your gut lacks these enzymes, this is when you can trigger symptoms of IBS.

Mono-Saccharides

This is a fructose that is found when a person has an excess amount of glucose in their diet. Our bodies need an equal amount of glucose in our system to stop any malabsorption. This means that while some of us can consume a certain amount of glucose, it is important to avoid foods that contain an excess amount. Some examples of these excessive foods include asparagus, honey, apples, and pears.

And Polyols

Polyols are also known as sugar alcohols. These can be found in a wide range of vegetables and fruits including sweet potatoes, mushrooms, pears, and apples. These sugar alcohols are also found artificial sweeteners in chewing gum, diabetic candy, and even protein powder. These polyols can only be partially absorbed into our small intestines. The rest continue into the large intestine, begin to ferment, and cause discomfort and bloating for some people.

As you begin to consider the low FODMAP diet, it is important to understand that one size does not fit all. This diet will change depending on your intolerance to certain foods. On the FODMAP diet, you will be following three different phases including: The Elimination Phase, The Reintroduction Phase, and the Maintenance Phase. We will go further into detail of each phase, so you have a full understanding before beginning.

The Elimination Phase

The Elimination phase is also known as the restriction phase. While this may seem intimidating, realize that this phase is only meant to last two to six weeks. This phase should only last long enough for you to gain control over your symptoms. Once this happens, you will move onto the reintroduction phase with the help of a professional. It is important that this stage is short as it can have long-term effects on your gut health.

To begin, you will want to create a personal list of foods you feel makes your IBS worse. If you are unsure which foods could be causing your symptoms, you will want to check out the next chapter to see an extended list of foods you should be avoiding. Some popular starters include chocolate, coffee, nuts, and certain fibers.

Once you have made your list, you will begin to eliminate these foods one at a time from your diet. It will take a couple of weeks before you notice any improvements. It does take some time for these foods to get through your system. However, if you do not notice any improvement, you will want to reintroduce these foods into your diet and try the next item on your list. Eventually, you will have a complete list of foods that trigger your IBS symptoms. Other popular foods to eliminate during this phase include: soy, gluten, and dairy products.

An important tool during this phase will be a food diary. This way, you will be able to keep track of which foods you are eating during the day, and any symptoms that may present themselves after they have been consumed. In general, the longer this phase is, the more likely you are to find that is triggering your IBS symptoms. It is important to remember that once eliminated, you will need to reintroduce foods slowly in the next phase.

The Reintroduction Phase

Once you have gone through your elimination period, you will be reintroducing these targeted foods back into your diet. While following the low FODMAP diet, you will need to introduce these foods back into your lifestyle one at a time.

As a tip for the reintroduction phase, we suggest starting on a Monday.

This way, you will be able to consume a small portion of the food, wait a few days, and see if you experience any symptoms. On day three, you can eat a larger portion and wait another couple days for any onset symptoms. Be sure to keep track of how you are feeling in your food diary so you can present it to a professional if need be. If you experience symptoms, this is a possible food trigger. If there is no symptom, you can assume that this certain food group is a good match for your diet.

After a while, you will have a complete list of foods that you need to assess, and you will start the elimination phase over again to double check. Once you eliminate and reintroduce, you will be able to create a diet you can stick with and eliminate any symptoms of IBS you may experience.

Maintenance Phase

While this may take time, the elimination and reintroduction phase are going to be very important while following the low FODMAP diet. These are going to be your tools in identifying foods that trigger your IBS symptom. The long-term goal is to create a wide variety of foods you can consume on a daily basis to ensure you are intaking all of your essential nutrients while eliminating the ones that make you feel lousy.

As you go through these phases, it is vital you listen to your body. Only you will be able to tell if you have a tolerance to certain foods. Remember that portion sizes will be important during these phases as well. While you may not react to small portions, larger portions may trigger the symptoms which you will want to avoid. The more tests you do, the more foods you will be able to add or subtract from your diet. While this may take some extra work, it will be worth it when you decrease your bloating and discomfort from IBS.

You may be wondering if you can follow this diet even if you have a certain lifestyle. Typically, the answer is yes! The only factor being that you could have a very limited number of foods allowed on your diet with any other limitations. Below, we will cover some of the more common diets and how you can also follow the low FODMAP diet as well!

Low FODMAP Diet with Vegan/Vegetarian Diet

If you follow a vegan or vegetarian diet, you may want to consider working with a dietary professional. Due to the fact you consume a diet that is different from most of the population, it can be more difficult to access foods that can work well with both diets. By working with a professional, they can ensure you still follow your diets without missing any essential nutrients your body needs.

While on the low FODMAP diet, it is important you keep re-testing foods. Remember that the elimination phase is meant to be short term. As you reintroduce old foods, you will be able to process if you can tolerate them or not. While you do this, you can find some staple foods, even if they happen to be high in FODMAPs.

If you follow a vegan or vegetarian diet, it will be vital that you pay special attention to your protein intake. As you will be learning later in the book, the low FODMAP diet includes a limitation of many legumes which may be a main source of protein for you right now. Instead of legumes, you can consider soy products or simply a smaller portion of legumes. Along with these switches, there are also milk substitutes to help with your protein intake. There is almond milk and other soy products to help out. Certain nuts and seeds also have varying levels of proteins for you to consider.

Low FODMAP Diet and Diabetes

If you have diabetes, you are most likely aware that there is no specific diabetic diet. In general, most people with diabetes follow a suggested balanced and healthy diet. If you wish to follow the low FODMAP diet while having diabetes, there are a few key rules you can follow to ensure you do not cause further harm to your health.

1. Planning

While on the low FODMAP diet, planning regular meals will be key. By doing this, you will be able to make sure that your blood glucose levels are always stable. By planning in advance, you can be successful in managing your diabetes while still following the low FODMAP diet. This stands especially true if you struggle finding healthy foods when you are away from your house. By being prepared, you will always have healthy options and can stay away from temptations. One good idea is to prep snacks for in-between your meals. These can be rice cakes, popcorn, or a simple fruit that is allowed in your low FODMAP diet.

2. Focus on Low FODMAP Carbohydrates

If you wish to follow the low FODMAP diet and eat healthy while having diabetes, eating starchy carbohydrates will be important for you. Some suitable options for you include wheat free bread, oats, potatoes, and rice. Before you include these, be sure to eliminate them from your diet to assure they are not triggers. Essentially, you will want to avoid any large portions of carbohydrates so you will be able to avoid any spikes in your blood glucose. You can do this by choosing slow-release carbohydrates like sweet potatoes or oats. On top of these carbs, you will also want to include allowed vegetables.

3. High Sugar Foods

As a person with diabetes, you already know that sugary foods cause your blood glucose levels to rise. On the low FODMAP diet, there is a low risk of consuming sugary foods such as soft drinks and cake, but they should still be avoided.

4. Low FODMAP Fruit

While fruits are a source of sugar, it will be important that you include a few portions of fruit per day. On the low FODMAP diet, there are plenty of options such as grapes, strawberries, bananas, and even oranges. You will want to pay special attention to your portion sizes as bigger portions, means higher amounts of fructose. You will also want to limit your portions of dried fruit, smoothies and fruit juices as they are typically pretty concentrated sources of fructose.

Low FODMAP Diet for Children

At this point, there has been very little research on the low FODMAP diet for children. Studies have shown that there are no real negative side effects for individuals who follow the low FODMAP diet for short period of time. However, if this diet were to carry on for longer than suggested, it could possibly have a negative effect on the gut flora balance in a child. If you are considering this diet for your child, there are several factors you will want to take into consideration.

First, your child will need to be seen by the pediatrician to confirm that your child has irritable bowel syndrome. Once it is diagnosed, the doctor will need to approve the diet and be carefully supervised to assure the safety of your child. Only after you follow these steps should you continue onto the elimination stage of the low FODMAP diet. For success on the diet, you can follow some of the following tips:

1. Inform Other Adults

Just like with any other diet restrictions, you will want to inform key adults of your child's restrictions. Whether it is a friend, a child care provider, or a teacher, this will be vital for the success of the diet. When these adults are in know of your child's diet, they will be able to address any stomach issues they may be having.

2. Involve Your Child

If your child is old enough, try to explain the diet to them in simple terms. You will want to explain that they are feeling sick due to the food they are eating. Be sure to include them and ask for their input in the food substitutions and menu. By making your child feel they are a part of the process, this may help your child comply with the new food rules.

3. Pack and Plan

Many parents fear diets for their children as they are always on the go! Luckily, the FODMAP diet is pretty easy to follow when you plan ahead. When you are at home, you most likely stock the fridge with low FODMAP foods. By planning ahead and packing your own snacks and lunches, you can assure your child will stick to the diet, so they do not make themselves sick.

4.   Forget the Small Stuff

Your kid is going to be a kid. If your child eats a restricted food every once in a while, it isn't going to ruin their diet altogether. Children typically do not have the self-discipline that adults have. They will most likely be tempted by restricted foods when at school or with their friends. You need to remember that while you want to stick to the diet most of the time, you can still allow your child some freedom when it comes down to what they are eating.

Exercise on the Low FODMAP Diet

While your diet may be causing your IBS symptoms, research has found that exercise can also help decrease any symptoms you may be suffering from. There are a few reasons why including regular moderate exercise will be important in the success of your diet.

First off, regular exercise can help reduce stress in your body. Typically, IBS tends to stress people out. When this happens, the nerves in your colon become tenser and can create abdominal pain. When your colon is tenser, this can slow down your bowel movements all together and cause constipation. A simple exercise such as cycling or walking can help release endorphins into your system and help release the tension in your colon. The more relaxed you are, the more flexible you will become.

Along with decreased stressed will come an increase of oxygen in your body. There are plenty of wonderful exercises such as tai chi and yoga that creates a breathing routine. When you take in these abdominal breaths, this helps increase the amount of oxygen in your body. As you increase oxygen, this will also help release any tension you are holding in your colon.

Finally, exercise can also increase your blood flow. As you begin to sweat, your body will be getting rid of toxins that could be creating discomfort in your colon. The more you sweat, the healthier you will be. Plus, the movement could help promote healthier bowel movements by moving blood to any problematic areas you may have.

As you consider exercise with your diet, remember that it will be vital to fuel your body before and after exercise. You will want to fuel about one to two hours before you work out. As long as it is included in your low FODMAP diet consider a banana with peanut butter or even oatmeal with some strawberries. The exercise can be any moderate activity of your choice from dancing, to running, to cycling, or even a little bit of strength training. Choose an exercise that makes you happy and one that you will stick with.

Reasons the Diet May Not Be Working

Speaking of sticking to a diet, some of you may follow these instructions and still suffer from IBS symptoms. If this still happens, you will want to take a look at your stress levels and the diet itself. While of course there is going to be a learning curve of the low FODMAP diet, allow yourself several weeks to change your food habits. Feel free to check back to the resources of this book to assure you are eating the foods allowed on the low FODMAP diet. If you still have no idea why you are experiencing the symptoms still, perhaps it is one of the following reasons that the diet isn't working:

1. Lack of Fiber

Fiber plays a very important role in keeping your stool regular. Often times, the low FODMAP diet will remove high fiber foods, which means you will need to pay special attention to your fiber intake. If you find yourself struggling, try speaking to a professional to find other options while on the low FODMAP diet. It will also be important that you drink plenty of water to move fiber through your system.

2. Too Much Fruit

While there are plenty of fruits on the low FODMAP diet, it is possible you are eating too much of it in one sitting. Typically, you will want to stick to only one serving at a time. If you want more fruit later in the day, try waiting two to three hours after the first one is consumed. As you practice this diet more, you will be able to tell your tolerance levels with the fruits so you can reduce that time in between servings.

3. Hidden FODMAPs

Often times, you could be consuming ingredients that are high in FODMAPs and have no idea. Typically, they are found in highly processed foods to help their taste and texture. FODMAPs are also found in some medications such as cough drops and cough syrup. Unfortunately, while they can help a cold, they are often high in sugar alcohols which can trigger your IBS symptoms. It will be important to read labels, which is included in the chapter to follow.

4. Portion Control

It is very easy to sit down and eat more than a portion. While on the low

FODMAP diet, allowed foods can become high FODMAPs when you exceed their allowed portion size. As an example, you may want to enjoy some rice cakes as a treat. A recommended serving size is only two rice cakes. If you eat double the allowed portion, this is when you may experience symptoms of IBS. Again, this is where reading labels carefully will come in handy while on the low FODMAP diet.

5. Stress

Stress is going to be a huge factor on the low FODMAP diet. If you are carefully following your diet, check your lifestyle. Stress itself can cause IBS symptoms so you may want to consider stress management skills along with a diet. You can try therapy or yoga. At the end of the day, your success is in your own hands.

If you continue to have IBS symptoms after following the diet and dealing with the issues from above, you may want to seek medical advice again. It is possible you have further intolerances that have not been explored yet. Also, the FODMAP diet will not work for everyone. If you have tried and failed, ask your doctor or dietician what the next step for you could be. For now, we will begin to cover the foods you can and cannot eat while on the low FODMAP diet.

Chapter 4: Low FODMAP diet foods

In the chapter to follow, you will find a list of both low and high FODMAP foods. As for the elimination phase, you will want to try to eliminate all of the high FODMAP foods. Once you are in the reintroduction stage, you will be able to introduce these foods back in order to see what is triggering your IBS symptoms.

As you choose your foods for your low FODMAP diet, remember that reading the ingredient list on a package is going to be vital for your diet success. Below, we will cover some of the basics of reading a food label. Too often, companies are able to hide food ingredients and could be triggering your symptoms without understanding why.

When you choose your foods, portion control will also be vital. When it comes to fruit, try your best to portion out one piece every few hours. As for processed foods, you will want to avoid them all together. If you ever have any doubts on low and high FODMAP foods, you can always revisit this chapter!

Reading and Understanding Nutrition Fact Label

If you are looking to eliminate certain foods from your diet, you will be surprised to learn that they can sneak into dishes without even realizing they are there. In order to stick with your diet, learning how to read and understand a nutrition fact label is going to be crucial for your diet.

A. Serving Size

When you first look at a label, you will want to check out the serving size along with the number of servings in any given package. These serving sizes are typically standardized so you can compare them to other similar foods. Remember that for some people, they can have smaller portions of FODMAP foods, but bigger portions could trigger IBS symptoms. When you are aware of a true serving size, this will make sticking to your diet a bit easier.

B. Calories

If you are on the low FODMAP diet to lose weight, this could be helpful for you. The calories in each package provide a measurement of how much energy comes in a serving of the food. The more calories you consume, the more you will gain weight. By being mindful of the calories in a portion, you will be able to manage your weight in a healthy manner.

C. Nutrients

When you look at a label, the first ones listed are typically the ones that Americans eat a good amount of. These can include Total Fat, Saturated Fat, Trans Fat, Cholesterol, and Sodium. While this isn't the main focus of the low FODMAP diet, it is something you should be mindful of for your general health.

D. Ingredients List

Finally, you will want to pay special attention to the ingredients list included on the package. If you are intolerant to certain ingredients, you will want to keep a food journal of these foods, so you always have them at hand to compare to a label. When looking at the ingredients list, they will be listed in order of weight from most to least. Eventually, you will know exactly what you can't eat and be able to compare easily in the store. As a beginner, remember to read the label of everything you put in your shopping cart.

When you understand the basics of reading a label, it is time to move onto learning the high and low FODMAP food list. We will begin with the high FODMAP foods. With this list, you will either want to avoid the foods altogether, or reduce them drastically. Of course, everyone's tolerances will be different but to help reduce any symptoms of IBS, you should reduce the following foods to enhance your health.

High FODMAP Foods (Avoid/ Reduce)

Fruits (High Fructose)

- Apples
- Avocado
- Apricots
- Blackcurrants
- Blackberries
- Boysenberry
- Currants
- Cherries
- Dates
- Figs
- Feijoa
- Guava
- Grapefruit
- Goji Berries
- Lychee
- Mango
- Nectarines
- Prunes
- Pomegranate
- Plums
- Pineapple
- Persimmon
- Pears
- Peaches
- Raisins
- Sultana
- Tamarillo
- Watermelon

Vegetables/ Legumes

- Asparagus
- Artichoke
- Butter Beans
- Broad Beans
- Black Eyed Peas
- Beetroot
- Bananas
- Baked Beans
- Choko
- Celery

- Cauliflower
- Cassava
- Fermented Cabbage
- Garlic
- Kidney Beans
- Leek
- Lima Beans
- Mushrooms

- Mixed Vegetables
- Pickled Vegetables
- Peas
- Red Kidney Beans
- Soy Beans
- Shallots
- Scallions
- Split Peas

Cereals and Grains

- Almond Meal
- Amaranth Flour
- Breadcrumbs
- Bread
- Biscuits
- Barley
- Bran Cereals
- Crumpets
- Croissants
- Cakes
- Cashews
- Cereal Bars
- Couscous
- Egg Noodles
- Freekeh

- Gnocchi
- Muesli Cereal
- Muffins
- Pastries
- Pasta
- Pistachios
- Udon Noodles
- Wheat Bran
- Wheat Cereals
- Wheat Flour
- Wheat Germ
- Wheat Noodles
- Wheat Rolls
- Spelt Flour

Sweeteners/ Condiments

- Agave
- Fruit Bar
- Fructose
- Hummus
- Honey
- High Fructose Corn Syrup
- Jam
- Molasses
- Pesto Sauce
- Relish
- Sugar-Free Sweeteners (Inulin, Isomalt, Lactitol, Maltitol, Mannitol, Sorbitol, Xylitol)
- Tahini Paste

Drinks

- Beer
- Coconut Water
- Fruit Juices (Apple, Pear, Mango)
- Kombucha
- Malted Drink
- Quinoa Milk
- Rum
- Soy Milk
- Soda
- Tea (Black Tea, Chai Tea, Dandelion Tea, Fennel Tea, Chamomile Tea, Herbal Tea, Oolong Tea)
- Whey Protein
- Wine

Dairy

- Cheese (Cream, Halloumi, Ricotta)
- Custard
- Cream

- Ice Cream/ Gelato

- Kefir

- Milk (Cow, Goat, Evaporated Milk, Sheep)

- Sour Cream

- Yogurt

While this may seem like a large list of foods you shouldn't eat, remember that ingredients will affect individuals a little differently. While you should limit the foods listed from above, it is okay to have them every once in a while. The point of this diet is to help reduce symptoms from IBS and bloating. At the end of the day, you are in charge of what you eat and understand how certain foods will make you feel.

Low FODMAP Foods

Fruits

- Ackee
- Breadfruit
- Blueberries
- Bilberries
- Bananas (Unripe)
- Clementine
- Cranberry
- Cantaloupe
- Carambola
- Dragon Fruit
- Guava (Ripe)
- Grapes
- Honeydew
- Kiwi Fruit
- Lime
- Lemon
- Mandarin
- Orange
- Plantain
- Papaya
- Passion Fruit
- Rhubarb
- Raspberry
- Strawberry
- Tangelo
- Tamarind

Vegetables

- Alfalfa
- Butternut Squash
- Brussel Sprouts
- Broccolini
- Broccoli
- Bok Choy
- Beetroot
- Bean Sprouts
- Bamboo Shoots
- Cucumber
- Courgette
- Corn

- Choy Sum
- Cho Cho
- Chives
- Chili
- Chick Peas
- Celery
- Carrots
- Cabbage
- Eggplant
- Fennel
- Ginger
- Green Pepper
- Green Beans
- Kale
- Leek Leaves
- Lentils
- Lettuce
- Olives
- Okra
- Pumpkin
- Peas (Snow)
- Parsnip
- Red Peppers
- Radish
- Sweet Potato
- Swiss Chard
- Sun-Dried Tomatoes
- Squash
- Spinach
- Spaghetti Squash
- Seaweed
- Scallions
- Turnip
- Tomato
- Water Chestnuts
- Yams
- Zucchin

Meat and Poultry

- Beef
- Chicken
- Deli Meats
- Lamb
- Prosciutto
- Pork
- Turkey
- Processed Meats

Seafood and Fish

- Fresh Fish (Cod, Haddock, Salmon, Trout, Tuna, Canned Tuna)

- Seafood (Crab, Lobster, Mussels, Oysters, Shrimp)

Breads, Cereals, Grains, and Nuts

- Bread
  Wheat Free
  Gluten Free
  Potato Flour
  Spelt Sourdough
  Rice
  Oat
  Corn
- Pasta
  Wheat Free
  Gluten Free
- Almonds
- Biscuit (Shortbread)
- Buckwheat (Noodles, Flour)
- Brazil Nuts
- Brown Rice
- Crackers

- Corn Tortillas
- Coconut Milk
- Cornflakes
- Corncakes
- Crispbread
- Corn Flour
- Chips (Plain)
- Mixed Nuts
- Millet
- Macadamia Nuts
- Oatcakes
- Oats
- Oatmeal
- Pretzels
- Potato Flour
- Popcorn
- Polenta

- Pine Nuts
- Pecans
- Rice

  White

  Rice

  Brown

  Basmati
- Rice Krispies
- Rice Flour
- Rice Crackers

- Rice Cakes
- Rice Bran
- Seeds

  Sunflower

  Sesame

  Pumpkin

  Poppy

  Chai
- Tortilla Chips
- Walnuts

Condiments, Sweets, and Sweeteners

- Almond Butter
- Acesulfame K
- Aspartame
- Chocolate

  White

  Milk

  Dark
- Erythritol
- Fish Sauce
- Glycerol
- Glucose
- Golden Syrup
- Jelly

- Ketchup
- Mustard
- Miso Paste
- Mayonnaise
- Marmite
- Marmalade
- Maple Syrup
- Oyster Sauce
- Peanut Butter
- Rice Malt Syrup
- Sucralose (Sugar)
- Stevia

- Sweet and Sour Sauce
- Shrimp Paste
- Saccharine
- Tomato Sauce
- Tamarind

- Vinegar
  Rice Wine Vinegar
  Balsamic Vinegar
  Apple Cider Vinegar
- Worcestershire Sauce
- Wasabi

Drinks

- Alcohol (Wine, Whiskey, Gin, Vodka, Beer)
- Coffee
- Chocolate Powder
- Protein Powder (Whey, Rice, Pea, Egg)
- Soya Milk
- Sugar-Free Soft Drinks
- Water

Dairy/ Eggs

- Butter
- Cheese (Swiss, Ricotta, Parmesan, Mozzarella, Goat, Fetta, Cottage, Cheddar, Camembert, Brie)
- Eggs
- Milk (Rice, Oat, Macadamia, Lactose-free, Hemp, Almond)
- Swiss Cheese
- Soy Protein
- Sorbet
- Tofu
- Tempeh
- Yogurt (Goat, Lactose-free, Greek, Coconut)

Herbs and Spices

- Bay Leaves
- Basil
- Curry Leaves
- Coriander
- Cilantro
- Fenugreek
- Lemongrass
- Mint
- Oregano
- Parsley
- Rosemary
- Sage
- Thyme
- Tarragon
- All Spice
- Black Pepper
- Chili Powder
- Cardamom
- Curry Powder
- Cumin
- Cloves
- Five Spice
- Fennel Seeds

- Nutmeg
- Saffron
- Turmeric
- Avocado Oil
- Coconut Oil
- Canola Oil
- Olive Oil
- Sesame Oil
- Sunflower Oil
- Soy Bean Oil
- Vegetable Oil
- Baking Soda
- Baking Powder
- Cocoa Powder
- Ghee
- Gelatin
- Lard
- Salt
- Yeast

As you can tell from the list from above, there are food choices for all different types of diets. Whether you are vegan, vegetarian, or follow a typical diet, there are plenty of choices for you.

The list from above may seem daunting, but as you learn your own version of the low FODMAP diet, you will be able to put together recipes from the ingredients you are allowed. The key to being successful on this diet is enjoying the foods you are allowed. Luckily in today's market, there are plenty of substitutes for ingredients that may trigger you. As long as you take the time to make this list, you will be able to make your new diet successful.

In the chapter to follow, we will be providing a couple different meal plans for you to follow. There will be a seven-day example vegan diet. Once you have read through this, you can move onto the fourteen-day low FODMAP starter diet. Remember that these are mere suggestions and you can make adjustments as needed.

Chapter 5: Low FODMAP Diet Meal plan

At this point in the book, you hopefully have a better understanding of the foods you can and cannot eat while on the low FODMAP diet. Before we jump into potential meal plans for you to follow, it is time to learn some delicious ingredients.

If you feel nervous about the diet due to the big list of foods to avoid, you absolutely shouldn't! Is your diet going to be different? Yes. However, when you are no longer experiencing diarrhea, constipation, bloating, and the other symptoms from IBS, you will be asking yourself why you didn't start sooner!

As you will find out from the recipes from below, there is a way to stick to your diet and enjoy your meal at the same time. You will find easy to make breakfast, lunch, and dinner recipes. Remember to pay special attention to the ingredients so you can determine if the recipe itself will stick within your own limits.

Low FODMAP Breakfast Recipes:

Small Banana Pancakes

Prep Time: Five Minutes

Cook Time: Twenty Minutes

Servings: Two

Portion: Four Mini Pancakes

Ingredients:

- Dairy-free Spread (Olive Oil) (3 T.)
- Ground Nutmeg (.25 t.)
- Ground Cinnamon (.50 t.)
- Salt (.125 t.)
- Baking Powder (.25 t.)
- Brown Sugar (1 T.)
- Gluten-free All-Purpose Flour (2 T.)
- Egg (2)
- Banana (2 Small, Unripe)

Instructions

1. Begin by heating a medium pan over medium heat before tossing in your dairy-free spread.
2. While this is cooking, go ahead and peel the banana before placing it into a bowl. Mash the banana until it becomes smooth and then add in the egg.
3. Once the egg and banana are mixed well, go ahead and add in the rest of the ingredients. At this point, you should have a mixture that resembles batter.
4. Spoon the mixture into your heated pan and cook the pancakes for a few minutes on each side or until they turn a nice golden color.
5. For extra flavor, try topping the pancakes with your favorite low FODMAP fruit!

Roasted Sausage and Vegetable Breakfast Casserole

Prep Time: Twenty-Five Minutes

Cook Time: Forty-Five Minutes

Servings: Eight

Ingredients:

- Eggs (12)
- Low FODMAP Milk (.50 C.)
- Dried Oregano (.50 t.)
- Salt and Pepper (.25 t.)
- Leek Tips (.50 C.)
- Red Bell Pepper (1)
- Lamb Sausage (1 Package)
- Baby Spinach (2 C.)
- Potato (1)
- Butternut Squash (1)
- Sweet Potato (1)
- Olive Oil (1 T.)

Instructions:

1. Before you begin prepping your food, you will want to preheat your oven to 400 degrees.
2. As your oven heats up, prepare the vegetables from the list above by peeling them and dicing the ingredients into bite-size pieces.

3. Once this is done, place the vegetables on a tray and drizzle them lightly with olive oil or a spread that is allowed on your own low FODMAP diet. Pop them into the heated oven for twenty minutes or until they are soft.

4. While the vegetables are cooking, you can cook your red bell pepper, leek, and sausage in a pan over medium heat. Be sure to cook all of these ingredients through.

5. Now that all of these ingredients are cooked, add in the vegetables to a large casserole dish.

6. In a small bowl, mix together the eggs and add in desired spices. When ready, gently pour the mix over the vegetables already placed in the casserole dish.

7. Place the dish in the oven for thirty minutes or until the eggs are set. This is a great dish to enjoy hot or cold for breakfast!

Blueberry Low FODMAP Smoothie

Prep Time: Five Minutes

Servings: One

Ingredients:

- Lemon Juice (1 t.)
- Maple Syrup (.50 T.)
- Rice Protein Powder (2 t.)
- Frozen Banana (1)
- Ice Cubes (6-10)
- Blueberries (20)
- Vanilla Soy Ice cream (.25 C.)
- Low FODMAP Milk (.50 C.)

Instructions:

1. Place all of the ingredients from above into a blender. Be sure to cut the frozen banana into smaller pieces.
2. Serve right away for a delicious breakfast.

Banana and Oats FODMAP Breakfast Smoothie

Prep Time: Five Minutes

Servings: One

Ingredients:

- Almond Milk (.50 C.)
- Linseeds (1 t.)
- Rolled Oats (1 T.)
- Banana (1)

Instructions:

1. Place all of the ingredients from above into a blender. Be sure you cut the banana into smaller pieces for easier blending.
2. Serve immediately for a filling and healthy meal.

Blueberry, Banana, and Peanut Butter Breakfast Smoothie

Prep Time: Five Minutes

Servings: One

Ingredients:

- Ice Cubes (6-10)
- Low FODMAP Milk (.75 C.)
- Blueberries (.50 C.)
- Peanut Butter (1 T.)
- Banana (.50)

Instructions:

1. Place all of the ingredients from above into a blender and blend until everything is smooth.
2. Serve immediately and enjoy!

Kale, Ginger, and Pineapple Breakfast Smoothie

Prep Time: Five Minutes

Servings: One

Ingredients:

- Ice (1 C.)
- Ginger (.25 T.)
- Kale (1 C.)
- Pineapple (.75 C.)
- Orange (.50)
- Low FODMAP Milk (1 C.)

Instructions:

1. Place all of the ingredients from above into a blender and blend until everything becomes smooth.
2. Serve immediately for a nice, healthy breakfast.

Strawberry and Banana Breakfast Smoothie

Prep: Five Minutes

Servings: One

Ingredients:

- Ice (1 C.)
- Maple Syrup (1 t.)
- Low FODMAP Milk (.75 C.)
- Strawberries (6)
- Banana (1)

Instructions:

1. Toss all of the ingredients into your blender and mix together until smooth.
2. Serve and for an extra treat, try adding some whipped cream!

Low FODMAP Soups and Salads:

Apple, Carrot, and Kale Salad

Prep Time: Ten Minute

Servings: Eight

Portion: .50 C.

Ingredients:

- Salt and Pepper (.25 t.)
- Maple Syrup (1.50 t.)
- Mustard (1 T.)
- Red Wine Vinegar (1.50 T.)
- Olive Oil (3 T.)
- Kale (.50 C.)
- Carrots (3)
- Apple (1 C.)

Instructions:

1. First step, you will want to create your dressing for the salad. You can do this by taking a small bowl and mixing together the maple syrup, mustard, vinegar, and oil. For some extra flavor, season with salt and pepper to taste.
2. Once this is done, take the kale, carrots, and apple and chop into fine, smaller pieces.
3. Finally, dress the salad, toss it a bit, and your meal is ready to be served!

Green Bean, Tomato, and Chicken Salad

Prep Time: Fifteen Minutes

Servings: Four

Portion: .50 C.

Ingredients:

- Lettuce (1 C.)
- Basil Leaves (2 T.)
- Cherry Tomatoes (10)
- Gruyere Cheese (.50 C.)
- Cooked Chicken (1 Lb.)
- Green Beans (.50 C.)

Instructions:

1. To begin, you will want to bring a medium pot of water to a boil. Once the water is boiling, cook your green beans for a few minutes. Once they are tender, drain the water from the pot and run the beans under cold water for a minute.
2. Next, take a large bowl and mix together all of the ingredients from above for a healthy salad.
3. For extra flavor, top your salad with any low FODMAP approved dressings.

Tuna Salad Low FODMAP Style

Prep Time: Five Minutes

Servings: Six

Portion: .50 C.

Ingredients:

- Salt and Pepper (to taste)
- Dried Dill (.50 t.)
- Lemon Juice (1.50 T.)
- Mayonnaise (.50 C.)
- Celery (.50)
- Tuna (2 Cans)

Instructions:

1. Start out by squeezing the liquid out of the tuna.
2. Once you have discarded the tuna, add it into a medium bowl with the vegetables from above.
3. When everything is stirred together, add in the dill, lemon juice, mayonnaise, along with the salt and pepper.
4. This mixture is great for any salad or sandwich!

Low FODMAP Pumpkin Soup

Prep Time: Ten Minutes

Cook Time: Fifteen Minutes

Servings: Six

Portion: 1 C.

Ingredients:

- Lactose-free Half and Half (.75 C.)
- Light Brown Sugar (1 T.)
- Canned Pure Pumpkin (1)
- Vegetable Soup Base (2 T.)
- Water (3 C.)
- Cayenne Pepper (.125 t.)
- Nutmeg (.25 t.)
- Cinnamon (.25 t.)
- Smoked Paprika (.25 t.)
- Scallions (.75 C.)
- Olive Oil (1 T.)
- Unsalted Butter (2 T.)
- Salt and Pepper to taste

Instructions:

1. To begin, you will want to heat up a medium sized pot over a low to medium heat. Once the pot is warm, you can add in your oil and butter until it begins to sizzle.

2. When the butter and oil are warm, add in your spices with the scallions and cook until they are soft.

3. Once this happens, add in the soup and water. Be sure to mix everything together before you add in the salt, brown sugar, and the canned pumpkin.

4. Now that these ingredients are placed in the pot, lower your heat and allow these to simmer for ten minutes or so. Feel free to stir every once in a while, to assure the ingredients are blended well.

5. Now, remove the soup from the heat and add in your half and half. Once the soup is cool, you can place the mixture into a blender and blend until it is smooth.

6. For extra flavor, season the soup with salt and pepper to taste.

Quinoa and Turkey Meatball Soup

Prep Time: Fifteen Minutes

Cook Time: Twenty Minutes

Servings: Eight

Portion: 1 C.

Ingredients:

- Collard Greens (5 C.)
- Celery (.50)
- Leek Tips (1 C.)
- Olive Oil (2 T.)
- Egg (1)
- Dried Basil (2 T.)
- Parsley (2 T.)
- Cooked Quinoa (.50 C.)
- Ground Turkey (1 Lb.)
- Turkey Stock (10 C.)
- Salt and Pepper to taste

Instructions:

1. To start out, you are going to want to make your meatballs for the soup. You will do this by taking a large mixing bowl and combine the egg, parsley, basil, quinoa, and turkey together. Gently take the mixture in your hands and form one inch balls.

2. Next, take a medium pan over medium heat and cook the turkey meatballs in olive oil for a few minutes. Be sure to flip the balls

over so that they are a nice golden-brown color all around.

3. Now that these are done, take a large pot over medium heat and add in a tablespoon of oil. Once the oil is sizzling, you can add in the leek and celery. Sauté these two ingredients for a minute before adding in the collard greens and stock.

4. When all of the ingredients are cooked, add in the meatballs and allow this mixture to simmer over a low heat for eight to ten minutes.

5. Remove the soup from the heat and allow to cool slightly before serving.

Mixed Vegetable, Bean and Pasta Soup

Prep Time: Fifteen Minutes

Cook Time: Thirty Minutes

Servings: Fourteen

Portion: .75 C.

Ingredients:

- Gluten-free Pasta (1 C.)
- Dried Thyme (1 t.)
- Smoked Paprika (1 t.)
- Dried Basil (1 t.)
- Zucchini (1)
- Squash (1)

- Bok Choy (2 C.)
- Carrots (3)
- Kale (1 C.)
- Red Potatoes (1 C.)
- Butternut Squash (1 C.)
- Crushed Tomatoes (1 Can)
- Water (8 C.)
- Leek Tips (.25 C.)
- Scallions (.75 C.)
- Olive Oil (2 T.)
- Salt and Pepper to taste

Instructions:

1. To start, you will want to take a large pot and begin to heat it over medium heat with the olive oil placed in the bottom.
2. Once the olive oil is sizzling, add in the leeks and scallions and allow them to cook until they become soft.
3. When these are ready, add in your prepared zucchini, squash, Bok choy, carrots, kale, potatoes, chickpeas, canned tomatoes, and the water. Season as desired and place the top on the pot.
4. Bring all of the ingredients from above to a boil and then turn the heat down to allow everything to simmer for at least thirty minutes. By the end, all of the vegetables should be tender.
5. While the soup cooks, you can cook the gluten-free pasta in another pot so by the end, you can combine everything and have a healthy meal!

Vegan Options:

Low FODMAP Coconut and Banana Breakfast Cookie

Prep Time: Ten Minutes

Cook Time: Twenty Minutes

Servings: Ten

Portion: One

Ingredients:

- Vanilla Extract (1 t.)
- Vegetable Oil (.25 C.)
- Maple Syrup (.25 C.)
- Banana (1)
- Baking Powder (.50 t.)
- Cinnamon (1 t.)
- Ground Flax Seeds (2 T.)
- Chia Seeds (2 T.)
- Unsweetened Coconut Flakes (.50 C.)
- Banana Chips (.50 C.)
- Gluten-free All-purpose Flour (.50 C.)
- Old-fashioned Oats (1 C.)

Instructions:

1. You will want to begin by heating your oven to 325 degrees.

2. While the oven heats up, take a medium bowl and mix together the baking powder, cinnamon, flax seeds, chia seeds, coconut flakes, banana chips, flour, and oats altogether.

3. In another bowl, mix together a mashed banana, vanilla, vegetable oil, and pale syrup. When both bowls are well combined, you can mix them together and begin to create your dough.

4. Next, take a greased cookie sheet and lay out balls of dough to create your cookies. When this is done, pop the cookie sheet in the oven for twenty minutes.

5. When the time is up, remove the cookies, allow to cool, and enjoy!

Lemon and Garlic Roasted Zucchini

Prep Time: Five Minutes

Cook Time: Twenty Minutes

Servings: Twelve

Portion: 1 C.

Ingredients:

- Olive Oil (1.50 T.)
- Zucchini (2)
- Lemon Zest (2 T.)
- Salt and Pepper to taste

Instructions:

1. You can begin by heating your oven to 425 degrees.
2. While this warms up, slice your zucchini into thin slices and place in a bowl with the lemon zest and olive oil. Assure it is covered completely before seasoning with salt and pepper.
3. Place the zucchini on a greased sheet pan and cook for twenty minutes.

Rainbow Low FODMAP Slaw

Prep Time: Ten Minutes

Servings: Twenty

Portion: 1 C.

Ingredients:

- Pomegranate Seeds (.50 C.)
- Carrots (3)
- Kale (1 C.)
- Red Cabbage (1 C.)
- Green Cabbage (1 C.)
- Lactose-free Yogurt (.50 C.)
- Dijon Mustard (1 t.)
- Sugar (2 T.)
- Apple Cider Vinegar (.25 C.)
- Canola Oil (.50 C.)

Ingredients:

1. Start out by creating your dressing for the slaw. You can do this in a small bowl, mix together the canola oil, apple cider vinegar, Dijon mustard, sugar, yogurt, and a little bit of salt.
2. In another bowl, toss together the different cabbage with the carrots and the kale.
3. Gently drizzle the dressing over the kale, and you have a delicious slaw that is full of color and flavor!

Vegan Roasted Red Pepper Farfalle

Prep Time: Ten Minutes

Cook Time: Ten Minutes

Servings: Four

Portion: 1 C.

Ingredients:

- Capers (.25 C.)
- Parsley (.75 C.)
- Olive Oil (.25 C.)
- Roasted Red Peppers (1 Jar)
- Gluten-free Farfalle Pasta (2 C.)

Instructions:

1. You can start this recipe by cooking your pasta according to the instructions on the side of the box.
2. Once the pasta is cooked through, drain the water and then place the pasta back into the pot.
3. Toss in the oil, parsley, roasted red peppers, and capers to the mixture.
4. Mix everything together and season with salt and pepper for extra flavor.

As you can tell, you can follow the low FODMAP diet and still enjoy delicious foods. While these are only some of the many recipes you can follow on your diet, there are plenty of resources out there to provide you with even more! With these resources in hand, we will now go over a simple seven and fourteen-day meal plan that is easy to follow.

With a limited food choices, you may be thinking to yourself that you are going to get bored quick. When it comes to a new diet, it is all about your frame of mind. On one hand, you could think negatively about it and return to your old eating habits. With choice, comes consequence. When you eat the foods that trigger you, you are going to feel lousy. Why make that choice when you can choose to eat healthy and feel better? Below, we will provide some simple meals for you to consider until you feel confident enough to create your own recipes

Breakfast Meal Plan Ideas:

- Eggs- Hard-boiled, over easy, or even scrambled. There are many ways to enjoy eggs!
- Lactose-Free Yogurt with any low FODMAP fruit
- Gluten-free Muffins
- Gluten-free French toast
- Gluten-free Oatmeal with cinnamon
- Rice Cereal with low FODMAP fruit
- Ground Turkey
- Smoothie with low FODMAP fruit

Lunch Meal Plan Ideas:
- Gluten-free Bread with Deli Meat and Cheese

- Chicken Noodle Soup
- Quinoa Bowl with low FODMAP Veggies or Grilled Chicken
- Salad
- Baked Potato with Lactose-free Butter

Dinner Meal Plan Ideas:

- Stir-Fried Rice
- Tacos
- Gluten-Free Pizza
- Grilled Chicken Salad
- Steak with Fresh Low FODMAP Vegetables
- Grilled Chicken with White Rice
- Rice Pasta with Marinara
- Snack Meal Plan Ideas:
- Rice Cakes with Peanut Butter
- Baby Carrots
- Lactose-free Yogurt
- Unripe Banana
- Unsalted Peanuts
- Pop Chips
- Gluten-free Pretzels
- Crackers with Cheese
- Hard-Boiled Egg

14- Day Meal Plan

Week One:

Meal	Monday	Tues.	Wed.	Thurs.	Friday
BFast	Small Banana Pancakes	Blueberry Smoothie	Roasted Sausage and Vegetable Breakfast Casserole	Strawberry and Banana Breakfast Smoothie	Banana and Oats FODMAP Breakfast Smoothie
Lunch	Apple, Carrot, and Kale Salad	Mixed Vegetable, Bean, and Pasta Soup	Low FODMAP Pumpkin Soup	Tuna Salad Low FODMAP Style	Quinoa and Turkey Meatball Soup
Dinner	Low FODMAP Veggie Latkes	Steak with Lemon and Garlic Roasted Zucchini	Left Over Mixed Vegetable, Bean, and Pasta Soup	Vegan Roasted Red Pepper Farfalle	Salad with Grilled Chicken and Homemade Dressing

Meal	Saturday	Sunday
Breakfast	Eggs and low FODMAP fruit	Rice Cereal with low FODMAP fruit
Lunch	Chicken Noodle Soup	Baked Potato with Lactose-free Butter
Dinner	Stir-Fried Rice	Gluten-free Pizza

Week Two:

Meal	Monday	Tuesday	Wednesday	Thursday	Friday
Breakfast	Gluten-free French Toast	Rice Cereal with low FODMAP fruit	Lactose-free Yogurt with low FODMAP fruit	Blueberry Smoothie	Small Banana Pancakes
Lunch	Quinoa Bowl	Salad with Approved Dressing	Gluten-free Sandwich with Deli Meat and Cheese	Mixed Vegetable, Bean, and Pasta Soup	Tuna Salad on Gluten-free Bread
Dinner	Grilled Chicken with White Rice	Grilled Chicken Salad	Salad with Approved Dressing	Gluten-free Tacos	Stir-Fried Rice

Meal	Saturday	Sunday
Breakfast	Smoothie with low FODMAP fruit	Lactose-free Yogurt with low FODMAP fruit
Lunch	Rice Pasta with Marinara	Chicken Noodle Soup
Dinner	Baked Potato with Lactose-free Butter	Grilled Chicken Salad

Vegan 7-Day Meal Plan

Meal	Monday	Tuesday	Wednesday	Thursday	Friday
Breakfast	Coconut Yogurt with Chia Seeds	Rice Cakes with Peanut Butter	Corn Flakes with Almond Milk	Gluten-free Bread with Almond Butter	Unripe Banana with Coconut Yogurt
Lunch	Lemon and Garlic Roasted Zucchini	Rainbow Low FODMAP Slaw with Gluten-free Bread	Vegan Roasted Red Pepper Farfalle	Low FODMAP Coconut and Banana Cookie with Coconut Yogurt	Salad with Approved Dressing
Dinner	Low FODMAP Veggie Latkes	Gluten-free Pasta with Approved Sauce	Plain Tempeh with low FODMAP Veggie of choice	Plain Tofu with Rice Noodles	Gluten-free Pizza with Soy Cheese

Meal	Saturday	Sunday
Breakfast	Blueberry Smoothie with Coconut Milk	Banana and Oat Smoothie with Coconut Milk
Lunch	Plain Tofu with Soba Noodles	Plain Tempeh with Gluten-free Pasta
Dinner	Grilled Cabbage Soup	Baked Brussel Sprouts with Plain Tofu

Chapter 6: Low FODMAP diet tips and tricks for success

Starting a new diet can be scary. As we said before, your frame of mind is going to be incredibly important. It is vital you think about your why when making food choices. Each meal, we have a chance to better our health; all it takes is a little thought behind each decision.

Of course, we want to see you succeed with your diet. Below, you will find a number of tips and tricks that have helped other clients on the low FODMAP diet. While some may work for you, others may not. You must adjust the low FODMAP diet to match your desired lifestyle so you not only stick with it but can enjoy it at the same time!

1. Read the Label

Reading the labels on packaged foods is going to be vital for the success of your diet. Unfortunately, many high FODMAP ingredients can have very confusing names. We suggest carrying a list of additives to avoid until you learn them by heart. When you are more aware, you can avoid the high FODMAP ingredients.

2. Water-soluble

In general, low FODMAP foods are going to be water-soluble, but this does not mean they are fat-soluble. If you are cooking a soup with an onion, you will want to take the onion out. Instead, try using onion-infused oils for the taste. It is quick fix that may help with your IBS triggers.

1. High Fructose Corn Syrup

High Fructose Corn Syrup is in everything. Again, it will be important that you learn how to read food labels so you will be able to avoid this mistake. This ingredient is in a number of foods including energy bars, juices, mayonnaise, frozen meals, and even popcorn. Check the label before you put anything into your shopping cart.

2. Fiber

If you pick up a product and it seems to have a high serving f fiber, you can assume it is due to a high FODMAP additive. Try to avoid any products that boast about their fiber; it's a trap! Any fiber additives will more than likely trigger your GI issues.

3. Onion and Garlic Powder

When it comes to choosing out your spices, pay special attention to the labels. You will want to avoid onion and garlic powders as they contain high FODMAPs. Luckily, there are plenty of delicious low FODMAP approved spices as you can find in the chapter from above.

4. "Natural"

If you find any frozen foods, brothers, or savory soups that claim they have "natural" flavors, go ahead and check out the label. You can assume that they contain garlic and onion, very popular IBS triggers. You will want to try your best to avoid these additives to your meals.

5. "Healthy"

As much as we would like to trust when products claim they are healthy, this does not equate to low FODMAP approved. Foods like asparagus and apples are supposedly "healthy" for you, but they can trigger IBS symptoms. As you go through the elimination process, you will learn just what you can and cannot eat and make the decision if something is healthy for you.

6. Beverages

Often times, people forget that beverages can contain FODMAPs. You will want to pay special attention to what you are putting into your body. If you ever have questions, feel free to refer to our lists in the chapter from above. Just because a beverage claims it has no net carbohydrates, this does not mean they aren't high in FODMAPs.

7. Portion Control

While you are on the low FODMAP diet, portion is going to be key to success. When you are reading labels, you will always want to pay special attention to portion size. While a low FODMAP diet is approved, a bigger portion may still trigger IBS symptoms. You will want to try your best to be mindful of portion control.

8. Learn About Yourself

As you start this diet, you will want to spend plenty of time on the elimination phase. The more you test, the more you will be able to figure out what foods you can and cannot eat. When you have more to choose from, you will be able to get more creative with your recipes. At the end of the day, only you know what is best for you. When you learn yourself, the diet will become that much easier.

9. Food and Meal Journal

Your food and meal journal are going to be an important tool for your low FODMAP diet journey. By keeping track of the foods, you can and cannot eat; it will make it easier when you go back to check out your history. We eat so many different types of foods through the day; it can be hard to remember which foods trigger you. By keeping a journal, it leaves little room for mistakes.

10. Use Your Fridge

If you are trying your best to stick with the low FODMAP diet, why leave anything up to chance? Do yourself a favor and take the time to remove any high FODMAP foods in your house. By keeping your pantry and fridge stocked with the low FODMAP foods you need, it deletes any temptations you may have in the house.

11. Have A Backup Plan

Dieting is hard, especially when you are first starting out. When you are planning out your meals, it is possible to miss one here or there. Try to stack your freezer with low FODMAP meals so you can cook them in a few minutes. When your first plan falls through, you will always have a backup. It is a win-win situation!

Chapter 7: Low FODMAP diet FAQ

As we are nearing our time together, hopefully, you are feeling better about starting the low FODMAP diet. While you have learned a lot about the diet, feel free to check back whenever you have a question about the diet. Whether you need a refresher on the benefits of the diet or a reminder of which foods you can and cannot eat, you will be able to find the information here easily.

To finish off, we will hopefully be able to answer any further questions you have about the low FODMAP diet. Simply remember that this diet is going to be specifically tailored up to you. Being diagnosed with IBS or other GI tract issues is not the end of the world. It will take some extra effort, but when your symptoms and discomfort are relieved, you will be thankful you made the choice to start the low FODMAP diet. For now, it is time to answer some more popular questions you may still have.

Q. I am following the low FODMAP diet and still experiencing symptoms, is this the right diet for me?

A. The answer could be yes and no. If you are following the diet and still find yourself with symptoms of IBS, there may be another culprit in your diet. Remember to keep a food diet with you at all times so you can find any triggers you may be missing.

Q. Can I follow the low FODMAP diet as a vegetarian?

A. Absolutely! You can follow this diet whether you are vegan or vegetarian, it will just take a little extra work. You will find in the chapters before there are plenty of choices, so long as the allowed foods are not triggers for your own body. Some good sources of protein for this diet would be chickpeas, tofu, tempeh, and more. If there is a will, there is always a way!

Q. How do I make sure I'm getting enough Fiber?

A. This is one of the bigger concerns for those following the low FODMAP diet, especially if constipation is an issue. Luckily, several good low FODMAP sources can help you keep your fiber intake up. These include chia seeds, brown rice, flax seeds, kiwi, oranges, white potato, rice bran and more. Check out the list provided in the fourth chapter for a longer list.

Q. Should I eat Larger or Smaller Meals on the Low FODMAP Diet?

A. In general, you should try to eat three main meals through your day and to snacks between these meals. If you are still hungry, you can always add in another snack. Remember that portion control is going to be vital while you are on the low FODMAP diet, so this is something you will want to keep in mind when plating your meals.

Q. What is the rule with fats and oils on the Low FODMAP Diet?

A. As a general rule, there are plenty of fats and oils that are low in FODMAPs. However, anything in excess can trigger IBS symptoms. You will want to be especially aware of any condiments or sauces that are oil-based such as salad dressings. Most of the time, these also include high FODMAPs like garlic. Remember to always read the labels before consuming anything. You can also refer to our extended grocery list to see which fats and oils are allowed on the diet.

Q. Can I eat meat on the low FODMAP Diet?

A. Yes and No. Some sources of animal protein such as fish and chicken are low in FODMAPs. However, if the meat is prepared already, you will want to avoid any additives that may trigger your symptoms. If you have any further questions, please refer to the food lists from the chapter above.

Q. What happens if I break my diet?

A. While the aim of the diet is to stick to it as much as possible, mistakes and slip ups will happen. Overall, you will want to achieve control over any symptoms you may be having. If you slip up, expect to experience the IBS symptoms. As long as you return to your diet, you will most likely be able to improve them in a few days.

Q. Is this a lifestyle?

A. No, the low FODMAP diet is not meant to last for a lifetime. The aim of the diet is to help heal your gut over a controlled period of time. This diet should only be followed for two to six weeks. After this, you can begin to introduce food back into your diet. This will change depending on each individual.

•

PART III

In this chapter, we are going to study the details of the reset diet and what recipes you can make.

Chapter 1: How to Reset Your Body?

Created by a celebrity trainer, Harley Pasternak, the body reset diet is a famous fifteen-day eating pattern that aims to jump-start weight loss. According to Pasternak, if you experience rapid loss in weight early in a diet, you will feel more motivated to stick to that diet plan. This theory is even supported by a few scientific studies (Alice A Gibson, 2017).

The body reset diet claims to help in weight loss with light exercise and low-calorie diet plans for fifteen days. The diet is divided into 3 phases of five days each. Each phase had a particular pattern of diet and exercise routine. You need to consume food five times every day, starting from the first phase, which mostly consists of smoothies and progressing to more solid foods in the second and third phases.

The three phases of the body reset diet are:

- **Phase One** – During this stage, you are required to consume only two snacks every day and drink smoothies for breakfast, lunch, and dinner.

In the case of exercise, you have to walk at least ten thousand steps per day.

- **Phase Two** – During this phase, you can eat two snacks each day, consume solid food only once, and have to replace any two meals of the day with smoothies. In case of exercise, apart from walking ten thousand steps every day, on three of the days, you also have to finish five minutes of resistance training with the help of four separate exercises.

- **Phase Three** – You can consume two snacks every day, but you have to eat two low-calorie meals and replace one of your meals with a smoothie. For exercise, you are required to walk ten thousand steps. Apart from that, you also have to finish five minutes of resistance training with the help of four separate exercises each day.

After you have finished the standard fifteen-day diet requirements, you have to keep following the meal plan you followed in the third phase. However, during this time, you are allowed to have two "free meals" twice a week in which you can consume anything you want. These "free meals" are meant as a reward so that you can avoid feeling deprived. According to Pasternak, depriving yourself of a particular food continuously can result in binge eating (Nawal Alajmi, 2016).

There is no official endpoint of the diet after the first fifteen days for losing and maintaining weight. Pasternak suggests that the habits and routines formed over fifteen days should be maintained for a lifetime.

Chapter 2: Science Behind Metabolism Reset

Several people take on a "cleanse" or "detox" diet every year to lose the extra holiday weight or simply start following healthy habits. However, some fat diet plans are often a bit overwhelming. For example, it requires a tremendous amount of self-discipline to drink only juices. Moreover, even after finishing a grueling detox diet plan, you might just go back to eating foods that are bad for you because of those days of deprivation. New studies issued in the *Medicine & Science in Sports & Exercise* shows that low-calorie diets may result in binge eating, which is not the right method for lasting weight loss.

Another research conducted by the researchers at Loughborough University showed that healthy, college-aged women who followed a calorie-restricted diet consumed an extra three hundred calories at dinner as compared to the control group who consumed three standard meals. They revealed that it was because they had lower levels of peptide YY (represses appetite) and higher levels of ghrelin (makes you hungry). They are most likely to go hog wild when you are feeling ravenous, and it's finally time to eat (Nawal Alajmi K. D.-O., 2016).

Another research published in *Cognitive Neuroscience* studied the brains of chronic dieters. They revealed that there was a weaker connection between the two regions of the brain in people who had a higher percentage of body fat. They showed that they might have an increased risk of getting obese because it's harder for them to set their temptations aside (Pin-Hao Andy Chen, 2016).

A few other studies, however, also revealed that you could increase your self-control through practice. Self-control, similar to any other kind of strength, also requires time to develop. However, you can consider focusing on a diet plan that can help you "reset" instead of putting all your efforts into developing your self-control to get healthy.

A reset is considered as a new start – one that can get your metabolism and your liver in good shape. The liver is the biggest solid organ of your body, and it's mainly responsible for removing toxins that can harm your health and well-being by polluting your system. Toxins keep accumulating in your body all the time, and even though it's the liver's job to handle this, it can sometimes get behind schedule, which can result in inflammation. It causes a lot of strain on your metabolism and results in weight gain, particularly around the abdomen. The best method to alleviate this inflammation is to follow a metabolism rest diet and give your digestive system a vacation (Olivia M. Farr, 2015).

Chapter 3: Recipes for Smoothies and Salads

If you want to lose weight and you have a particular period within which you want to achieve it, then here are some recipes that are going to be helpful.

Green Smoothie

Total Prep & Cooking Time: 2 minutes

Yields: 1 serving

Nutrition Facts: Calories: 144 | Carbs: 28.2g | Protein: 3.4g | Fat: 2.9g | Fiber: 4.8g

Ingredients:

- One cup each of
  - o Almond milk
  - o Raw spinach
- One-third of a cup of strawberries
- One orange, peeled

Method:

1. Add the peeled orange, strawberries, almond milk, and raw spinach in a blender and blend everything until you get a smooth paste. You can add extra water if required to achieve the desired thickness.

2. Pour out the smoothie into a glass and serve.

Strawberry Banana Smoothie

Total Prep & Cooking Time: 5 minutes

Yields: 2 servings

Nutrition Facts: Calories: 198| Carbs: 30.8g | Protein: 5.9g | Fat: 7.1g | Fiber: 4.8g

Ingredients:

- Half a cup each of
  - Milk
  - Greek yogurt
- One banana, frozen and quartered
- Two cups of fresh strawberries, halved

Method:

1. Add the milk, Greek yogurt, banana, and strawberries into a high-powered blender and blend until you get a smooth mixture.

2. Pour the smoothie equally into two separate glasses and serve.

Notes:

- *Don't add ice to the smoothie as it can make it watery very quickly. Using frozen bananas will keep your smoothie cold.*

- *As you're using bananas and strawberries, there is no need to add any artificial sweetener.*

Salmon Citrus Salad

Total Prep & Cooking Time: 20 minutes

Yields: 6 servings

Nutrition Facts: Calories: 336 | Carbs: 20g | Protein: 17g | Fat: 21g | Fiber: 5g

Ingredients:

- One pound of Citrus Salmon (slow-roasted)
- Half of an English cucumber, sliced
- One tomato (large), sliced into a quarter of an inch thick pieces
- One grapefruit, peeled and cut into segments
- Two oranges, peeled and cut into segments
- Three beets, roasted and quartered
- One avocado
- Boston lettuce leaves
- Two tablespoons of red wine vinegar
- Half of a red onion
- Flakey salt
- Aleppo pepper flakes

For the Citrus Shallot Vinaigrette,

- Five tablespoons of olive oil (extra-virgin)
- One clove of garlic, smashed
- Salt and pepper
- One and a half tablespoons of rice wine vinegar
- Two tablespoons of orange juice or fresh lemon juice

- One tablespoon of shallot, minced

Method:

For preparing the Citrus Shallot Vinaigrette.

1. Add the ingredients for the vinaigrette in a bowl and whisk them together.

2. Keep the mixture aside.

For assembling the salad,

1. Add the onions and vinegar in a small bowl and pickle them by letting them sit for about fifteen minutes.

2. In the meantime, place the lettuce leaves on the serving plate.

3. Dice the avocado in half and eliminate the pit. Then scoop the flesh and add them onto the plate. Sprinkle a dash of flakey salt and Aleppo pepper on top to season it.

4. Add the quartered beets onto the serving plate along with the grapefruit and orange segments.

5. Salt the cucumber and tomato slices lightly and add them onto the plate.

6. Then, scatter the pickled onions on top and cut the salmon into bits and add it on the plate.

7. Lastly, drizzle the Citrus Shallot Vinaigrette on top of the salad and finish off with a dash of flakey salt.

Chapter 4: Quick and Easy Breakfast and Main Course Recipes

Quinoa Salad

Total Prep & Cooking Time: 40 minutes

Yields: Eight servings

Nutrition Facts: Calories: 205 | Carbs: 25.9g | Protein: 6.1g | Fat: 9.4g | Fiber: 4.6g

Ingredients:

- One tablespoon of red wine vinegar
- One-fourth of a cup each of
  - Lemon juice (about two to three lemons)
  - Olive oil
- One cup each of
  - Quinoa (uncooked), rinsed with the help of a fine-mesh colander
  - Flat-leaf parsley (from a single large bunch), finely chopped
- Three-fourth of a cup of red onion (one small red onion), chopped
- One red bell pepper (medium-sized), chopped
- One cucumber (medium-sized), seeded and chopped
- One and a half cups of chickpeas (cooked), or One can of chickpeas (about fifteen ounces), rinsed and drained
- Two cloves of garlic, minced or pressed
- Two cups of water
- Black pepper, freshly ground
- Half a teaspoon of fine sea salt

Method:

1. Place a medium-sized saucepan over medium-high heat and add the rinsed quinoa into it along with the water. Allow the mixture to boil and then reduce the heat and simmer it. Cook for about fifteen minutes so that the quinoa has absorbed all the water. As time goes on, decrease the heat and maintain a gentle simmer. Take the saucepan away from the heat and cover it with a lid. Allow the cooked quinoa to rest for about five minutes to give it some time to increase in size.

2. Add the onions, bell pepper, cucumber, chickpeas, and parsley in a large serving bowl and mix them together. Keep the mixture aside.

3. Add the garlic, vinegar, lemon juice, olive oil, and salt in another small bowl and whisk the ingredients so that they are appropriately combined. Keep this mixture aside.

4. When the cooked quinoa has almost cooled down, transfer it to the serving bowl. Add the dressing on top and toss to combine everything together.

5. Add an extra pinch of sea salt and the black pepper to season according to your preference. Allow the salad to rest for five to ten minutes before serving it for the best results.

6. You can keep the salad in the refrigerator for up to four days. Make sure to cover it properly.

7. You can serve it at room temperature or chilled.

Notes: Instead of cooking additional quinoa, you can use about three cups of leftover quinoa for making this salad. Moreover, you can also serve this salad with fresh greens and an additional drizzle of lemon juice and olive oil. You can also add a dollop of cashew sour cream or crumbled feta cheese as a topping.

Herb and Goat Cheese Omelet

Total Prep & Cooking Time: 20 minutes

Yields: Two servings

Nutrition Facts: Calories: 233 | Carbs: 3.6g | Protein: 16g | Fat: 17.6g | Fiber: 1g

Ingredients:

- Half a cup each of
  - Red bell peppers (3 x quarter-inch), julienne-cut
  - Zucchini, thinly sliced
- Four large eggs
- Two teaspoons of olive oil, divided
- One-fourth of a cup of goat cheese (one ounce), crumbled
- Half a teaspoon of fresh tarragon, chopped
- One teaspoon each of
  - Fresh parsley, chopped
  - Fresh chives, chopped
- One-eighth of a teaspoon of salt
- One-fourth of a teaspoon of black pepper, freshly ground (divided)
- One tablespoon of water

Method:

1. Break the eggs into a bowl and add one tablespoon of water into it. Whisk them together and add in one-eighth of a teaspoon each of salt and ground black pepper.

2. In another small bowl, mix the goat cheese, tarragon, and parsley and keep it aside.

3. Place a nonstick skillet over medium heat and heat one teaspoon of olive oil in it. Add in the sliced zucchini, bell pepper, and the remaining one-eighth of a teaspoon of black pepper along with a dash of salt. Cook for about four minutes so that the bell pepper and zucchini get soft. Transfer the zucchini-bell pepper mixture onto a plate and cover it with a lid to keep it warm.

4. Add about half a teaspoon of oil into a skillet and add in half of the whisked egg into it. Do not stir the eggs and let the egg set slightly. Loosen the set edges of the omelet carefully with the help of a spatula. Tilt the skillet to move the uncooked part of the egg to the side. Keep following this method for about five seconds so that there is no more runny egg in the skillet. Add half of the crumbled goat cheese mixture evenly over the omelet and let it cook for another minute so that it sets.

5. Transfer the omelet onto a plate and fold it into thirds.

6. Repeat the process with the rest of the egg mixture, half a teaspoon of olive oil, and the goat cheese mixture.

7. Add the chopped chives on top of the omelets and serve with the bell pepper and zucchini mixture.

Mediterranean Cod

Total Prep & Cooking Time: 15 minutes

Yields: 4 servings

Nutrition Facts: Calories: 320 | Carbs: 31g | Protein: 35g | Fat: 8g | Fiber: 8g

Ingredients:

- One pound of spinach
- Four fillets of cod (almost one and a half pounds)
- Two zucchinis (medium-sized), chopped
- One cup of marinara sauce
- One-fourth of a teaspoon of red pepper, crushed
- Two cloves of garlic, chopped
- One tablespoon of olive oil
- Salt and pepper, according to taste
- Whole wheat roll, for serving

Method:

1. Place a ten-inch skillet on medium heat and add the marinara sauce and zucchini into it. Combine them together and let it simmer on medium heat.

2. Add the fillets of cod into the simmering sauce. Add one-fourth of a teaspoon each of salt and pepper too. Cover the skillet with a lid and let it cook for about seven minutes so that the cod gets just opaque throughout.

3. In the meantime, place a five-quart saucepot on medium heat and heat the olive oil in it. Add in the crushed red pepper and minced garlic. Stir and cook for about a minute.

4. Then, add in the spinach along with one-eighth of a teaspoon of salt. Cover the saucepot with a lid and let it cook for about five minutes, occasionally stirring so that the spinach gets wilted.

5. Add the spinach on the plates and top with the sauce and cod mixture and serve with the whole wheat roll.

Grilled Chicken and Veggies

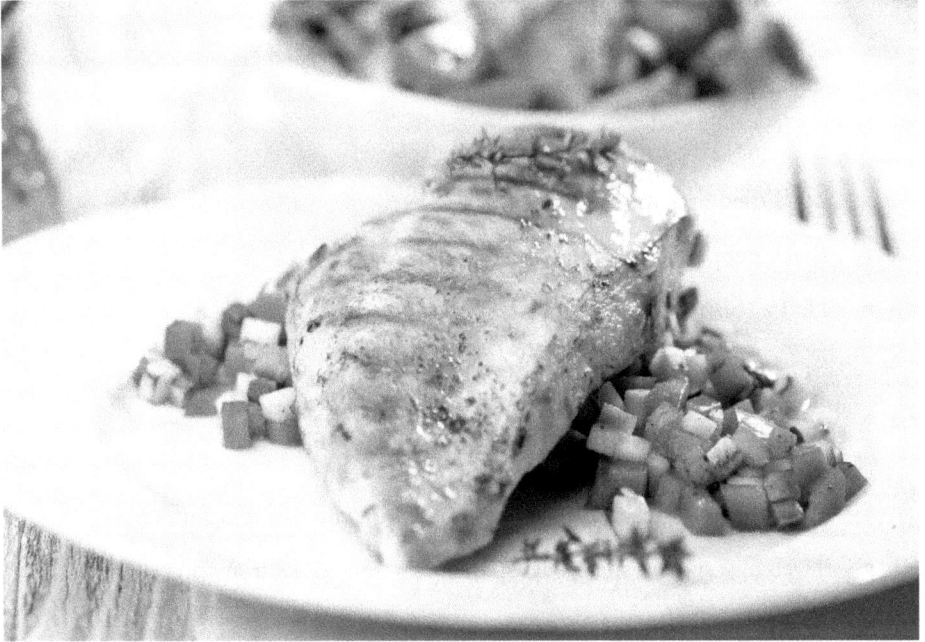

Total Prep & Cooking Time: 35 minutes

Yields: 4 servings

Nutrition Facts: Calories: 305 | Carbs: 11g | Protein: 26g | Fat: 17g | Fiber: 3g

Ingredients:

For the marinade,

- Four cloves of garlic, crushed

- One-fourth of a cup each of
  - Fresh lemon juice
  - Olive oil
- One teaspoon each of
  - Salt
  - Smoked paprika
  - Dried oregano
- Black pepper, according to taste
- Half a teaspoon of red chili flakes

For the grilling,

- Two to three zucchinis or courgette (large), cut into thin slices
- Twelve to sixteen spears of asparagus, woody sides trimmed
- Broccoli
- Two bell peppers, seeds eliminated and cut into thin slices
- Four pieces of chicken breasts (large), skinless and de-boned

Method:

1. Preheat your griddle or grill pan.

2. Sprinkle some salt on top of the chicken breasts to season them. Keep them aside to rest while you prepare the marinade.

3. For the marinade, mix all the ingredients properly.

4. Add about half of the marinade over the vegetables and the other half over the seasoned chicken breasts. Allow the marinade to rest for a couple of minutes.

5. Place the chicken pieces on the preheated grill. Grill for about five to seven minutes on each side until they are cooked according to your preference. The time on the grill depends on the thickness of the chicken breasts.

6. Remove them from the grill and cover them using a foil. Set it aside to rest and prepare to grill the vegetables in the meantime.

7. Grill the vegetables for a few minutes until they begin to char and are crispy yet tender.

8. Remove them from the grill and transfer them onto a serving plate. Serve the veggies along with the grilled chicken and add the lemon wedges on the side for squeezing.

Notes: *You can add as much or as little vegetables as you like. The vegetable amounts are given only as a guide. Moreover, feel free to replace some of them with the vegetables you like to eat.*

Stuffed Peppers

Total Prep & Cooking Time: 50 minutes

Yields: 4 servings

Nutrition Facts: Calories: 438 | Carbs: 32g | Protein: 32g | Fat: 20g | Fiber: 5g

Ingredients:

For the stuffed peppers,

- One pound of ground chicken or turkey
- Four bell peppers (large) of any color
- One and a quarter of a cups of cheese, shredded
- One and a half cups of brown rice, cooked (you can use cauliflower rice or quinoa)
- One can (about fourteen ounces) of fire-roasted diced tomatoes along with its juices
- Two teaspoons of olive oil (extra-virgin)
- One teaspoon each of
  - Garlic powder
  - Ground cumin
- One tablespoon of ground chili powder
- One-fourth of a teaspoon of black pepper
- Half a teaspoon of kosher salt

For serving,

- Sour cream or Greek yogurt

- Salsa

- Freshly chopped cilantro

- Avocado, sliced

- Freshly squeezed lemon juice

Method:

1. Preheat your oven to 375 degrees Fahrenheit.

2. Take a nine by thirteen-inch baking dish and coat it lightly with a nonstick cooking spray.

3. Take the bell peppers and slice them from top to bottom into halves. Remove the membranes and the seeds. Keep the bell peppers in the baking dish with the cut-side facing upwards.

4. Place a large, nonstick skillet on medium-high heat and heat the olive oil in it. Add in the chicken, pepper, salt, garlic powder, ground cumin, and chili powder and cook for about four minutes so that the chicken is cooked through and gets brown. Break apart the chicken while it's cooking. Drain off any excess liquid and then add in the can of diced tomatoes along with the juices. Allow it to simmer for a minute.

5. Take the pan away from the heat. Add in the cooked rice along with three-fourth of a cup of the shredded cheese and stir everything together.

6. Add this filling inside the peppers and add the remaining shredded cheese as a topping.

7. Add a little amount of water into the pan containing the peppers so that it barely covers the bottom of the pan.

8. Keep it uncovered and bake it in the oven for twenty-five to thirty-five minutes so that the cheese gets melted and the peppers get soft.

9. Add any of your favorite fixings as a topping and serve hot.

Notes:

- *For preparing the stuffed peppers ahead of time, make sure to allow the rice and chicken mixture to cool down completely before filling the peppers. You can prepare the stuffed peppers before time, and then you have to cover it with a lid and keep it in the refrigerator for a maximum of twenty-four hours before baking the peppers.*

- *If you're planning to reheat the stuffed peppers, gently reheat them in your oven or microwave. If you're using a microwave for this purpose, make sure to cut the peppers into pieces to warm them evenly.*

- *You can store any leftovers in the freezer for up to three months. Alternatively, you can keep them in the refrigerator for up to four days. Allow it to thaw in the fridge overnight.*

Brussels Sprouts With Honey Mustard Chicken

Total Prep & Cooking Time: Fifty minutes

Yields: Four servings

Nutrition Facts: Calories: 360 | Carbs: 14.5g | Protein: 30.8g | Fat: 20g | Fiber: 3.7g

Ingredients:

- One and a half pounds of Brussels sprouts, divided into two halves
- Two pounds of chicken thighs, skin-on and bone-in (about four medium-sized thighs)
- Three cloves of garlic, minced
- One-fourth of a large onion, cut into slices
- One tablespoon each of
  - Honey
  - Whole-grain mustard
  - Dijon mustard
- Two tablespoons of freshly squeezed lemon juice (one lemon)
- One-fourth of a cup plus two tablespoons of olive oil (extra-virgin)
- Freshly ground black pepper
- Kosher salt
- Non-stick cooking spray

Method:

1. Preheat your oven to 425 degrees Fahrenheit.

2. Take a large baking sheet and grease it with nonstick cooking spray. Keep it aside.

3. Add the minced garlic, honey, whole-grain mustard, Dijon mustard, one tablespoon of the lemon juice, one-fourth cup of the olive oil in a medium-sized bowl and mix them together. Add the Kosher salt and black pepper to season according to your preference.

4. Dip the chicken thighs into the sauce with the help of tongs and coat both sides. Transfer the things on the baking sheet. You can get rid of any extra sauce.

5. Mix the red onion and Brussels sprouts in a medium-sized bowl and drizzle one tablespoon of lemon juice along with the remaining two tablespoons of olive oil onto it. Toss everything together until the vegetables are adequately coated.

6. Place the red onion-Brussels sprouts mixture on the baking sheet around the chicken pieces. Ensure that the chicken and vegetables are not overlapping.

7. Sprinkle a little amount of salt and pepper on the top and keep it in the oven to roast for about thirty to thirty-five minutes so that the Brussels sprouts get crispy and the chicken has an internal temperature of 165 degrees Fahrenheit and has turned golden brown.

8. Serve hot.

Quinoa Stuffed Chicken

Total Prep & Cooking Time: 50 minutes

Yields: Four servings

Nutrition Facts: Calories: 355 | Carbs: 28g | Protein: 30g | Fat: 13g | Fiber: 4g

Ingredients:

- One and a half cups of chicken broth
- Three-fourths of a cup of quinoa (any color of your choice)
- Four chicken breasts (boneless and skinless)
- One lime, zested and one tablespoon of lime juice
- One-fourth of a cup of cilantro, chipped
- One-third of a cup of unsweetened coconut, shaved or coconut chips
- One Serrano pepper, seeded and diced
- Two cloves of garlic, minced
- Half a cup of red onion, diced
- Three-fourth of a cup of bell pepper, diced
- One tablespoon of coconut oil
- One teaspoon each of
  - Salt
  - Chili powder
  - Ground cumin

Method:

1. Preheat your oven to 375 degrees Fahrenheit.

2. Take a rimmed baking sheet and line it with parchment paper.

3. Place a medium-sized saucepan over medium-high heat and add the coconut oil in it. After it has melted, add in the Serrano peppers, garlic, red onion, and bell pepper and sauté for about one to two minutes so that they soften just a bit. Make sure that the vegetables are still bright in color. Then transfer the cooked vegetables into a bowl.

4. Add the quinoa in the empty sauce pot and increase the heat to high. Pour the chicken broth in it along with half a teaspoon of salt. Close the lid of the pot and bring it to a boil, allowing the quinoa to cook for about fifteen minutes so that the surface of the quinoa develops vent holes, and the broth has absorbed completely. Take the pot away from the heat and allow it to steam for an additional five minutes.

5. In the meantime, cut a slit along the long side in each chicken breast. It will be easier with the help of a boning knife. You are making a deep pocket in each breast, having a half-inch border around the remaining three attached sides. Keep the knife parallel to the cutting board and cut through the middle of the breast and leaving the opposite side attached. Try to cut it evenly as it's challenging to cook thick uncut portions properly in the oven. After that, add salt, cumin, and chili powder on all sides of the chicken.

6. When the quinoa has turned fluffy, add in the lime juice, lime zest, shaved coconut, and sautéed vegetables and stir them in. Taste the mixture and adjust the salt as per your preference.

7. Add the confetti quinoa mixture inside the cavity of the chicken breast. Place the stuffed breasts on the baking sheet with the quinoa facing upwards. They'll look like open envelopes.

8. Bake them in the oven for about twenty minutes.

9. Serve warm.

Kale and Sweet Potato Frittata

Total Prep & Cooking Time: 30 minutes

Yields: 4 servings

Nutrition Facts: Calories: 144 | Carbs: 10g | Protein: 7g | Fat: 9g | Fiber: 2g

Ingredients:

- Three ounces of goat cheese
- Two cloves of garlic
- Half of a red onion (small)
- Two cups each of
  - Sweet potatoes
  - Firmly packed kale, chopped
- Two tablespoons of olive oil
- One cup of half-and-half
- Six large eggs
- Half a teaspoon of pepper, freshly ground
- One teaspoon of Kosher salt

Method:

1. Preheat your oven to 350 degrees Fahrenheit.

2. Add the eggs, half-and-half, salt, and black pepper in a bowl and whisk everything together.

3. Place a ten-inch ovenproof nonstick skillet over medium heat and add one tablespoon of oil in it. Sauté the sweet potatoes in the skillet for about eight to ten minutes so that they turn soft and golden brown. Transfer them onto a plate and keep warm.

4. Next, add in the remaining one tablespoon of oil and sauté the kale along with the red onions and garlic in it for about three to four minutes so that the kale gets soft and wilted. Then, add in the whisked egg mixture evenly over the vegetables and cook for an additional three minutes.

5. Add some goat cheese on the top and bake it in the oven for ten to fourteen minutes so that it sets.

Walnut, Ginger, and Pineapple Oatmeal

Total Prep & Cooking Time: 30 minutes

Yields: 4 servings

Nutrition Facts: Calories: 323 | Carbs: 61g | Protein: 6g | Fat: 8g | Fiber: 5g

Ingredients:

- Two large eggs
- Two cups each of
  - Fresh pineapple, coarsely chopped
  - Old-fashioned rolled oats
  - Whole milk
- One cup of walnuts, chopped

- Half a cup of maple syrup

- One piece of ginger

- Two teaspoons of vanilla extract

- Half a teaspoon of salt

Method:

1. Preheat your oven to 400 degrees Fahrenheit.

2. Add the ginger, walnuts, pineapple, oats, and salt in a large bowl and mix them together. Add the mixture evenly among four ten-ounce ramekins and keep them aside.

3. Whisk the eggs along with the milk, maple syrup, and vanilla extract in a medium-sized bowl. Pour one-quarter of this mixture into each ramekin containing the oat-pineapple mixture.

4. Keep the ramekins on the baking sheet and bake them in the oven for about twenty-five minutes until the oats turn light golden brown on the top and have set properly.

5. Serve with some additional maple syrup on the side.

Caprese Salad

Total Prep & Cooking Time: 15 minutes

Yields: 4 servings

Nutrition Facts: Calories: 216 | Carbs: 4g | Protein: 13g | Fat: 16g | Fiber: 1g

Ingredients:

For the salad,

- Nine basil leaves (medium-sized)
- Eight ounces of fresh whole-milk mozzarella cheese
- Two tomatoes (medium-sized)
- One-fourth of a teaspoon of black pepper, freshly ground
- Half a teaspoon of Kosher salt, or one-fourth of a teaspoon of sea salt

For the dressing,

- One teaspoon of Dijon mustard
- One tablespoon each of
  - Balsamic vinegar
  - Olive oil

Method:

1. Add the olive oil, balsamic vinegar, and Dijon mustard into a small bowl and whisk them together with the help of a small hand whisk so that you get a smooth salad dressing. Keep it aside.

2. Cut the tomatoes into thin slices and try to get ten slices in total.

3. Cut the mozzarella into nine thin slices with the help of a sharp knife.

4. Place the slices of tomatoes and mozzarella on a serving plate, alternating and overlapping one another. Then, add the basil leaves on the top.

5. Season the salad with black pepper and salt and drizzle the prepared dressing on top.

6. Serve immediately.

One-Pot Chicken Soup

Total Prep & Cooking Time: 30 minutes

Yields: 6 servings

Nutrition Facts: Calories: 201 | Carbs: 20g | Protein: 16g | Fat: 7g | Fiber: 16g

Ingredients:

- Three cups of loosely packed chopped kale (or other greens of your choice)
- Two cups of chicken, shredded
- One can of white beans (about fifteen ounces), slightly drained
- Eight cups of broth (vegetable broth or chicken broth)
- Four cloves of garlic, minced
- One cup of yellow or white onion, diced
- One tablespoon of avocado oil (skip if you are using bacon)
- One strip of uncured bacon, chopped (optional)
- Black pepper + sea salt, according to taste

Method:

1. Place a Dutch oven or a large pot over medium heat. When it gets hot, add in the oil or bacon (optional), stirring occasionally, and allow it to get hot for about a minute.

2. Then, add in the diced onion and sauté for four to five minutes, occasionally stirring so that the onions get fragrant and translucent. Add in the minced garlic next and sauté for another two to three minutes. Be careful so as not to burn the ingredients.

3. Then, add the chicken, slightly drained white beans, and broth and bring the mixture to a simmer. Cook for about ten minutes to bring out all the flavors. Taste the mixture and add salt and pepper to season according to your preference. Add in the chopped kale in the last few minutes of cooking. Cover the pot and let it cook until the kale has wilted.

4. Serve hot.

Notes: You can store any leftovers in the freezer for up to a month. Or, you can store them in the refrigerator for a maximum of three to four days. Simply reheat on the stovetop or in the microwave and eat it later.

Chocolate Pomegranate Truffles

Total Prep & Cooking Time: 10 minutes

Yields: Twelve to Fourteen truffles

Nutrition Facts: Calories: 95 | Carbs: 26g | Protein: 1g | Fat: 2g | Fiber: 3g

Ingredients:

- One-third of a cup of pomegranate arils
- Half a teaspoon each of
  - Vanilla extract
  - Ground cinnamon
- Half a cup of ground flax seed
- Two tablespoons of cocoa powder (unsweetened)
- About one tablespoon of water
- One and a half cups of pitted Medjool dates
- One-eighth of a teaspoon of salt

Method:

1. Add the pitted dates in a food processor and blend until it begins to form a ball. Add some water and pulse again. Add in the vanilla, cinnamon, flax seeds, cocoa powder, and salt and blend until everything is combined properly.

2. Turn off the food processor and unplug it. Add in the pomegranate arils and fold them in the mixture so that they are distributed evenly.

3. Make twelve to fourteen balls using the mixture. You can create an outer coating or topping if you want by rolling the balls in finely shredded coconut or cocoa powder.

Notes: *You can store the chocolate pomegranate truffles in the fridge in an air-tight container for a maximum of three days.*

PART IV

Chapter 1: Tasty Breakfast Options

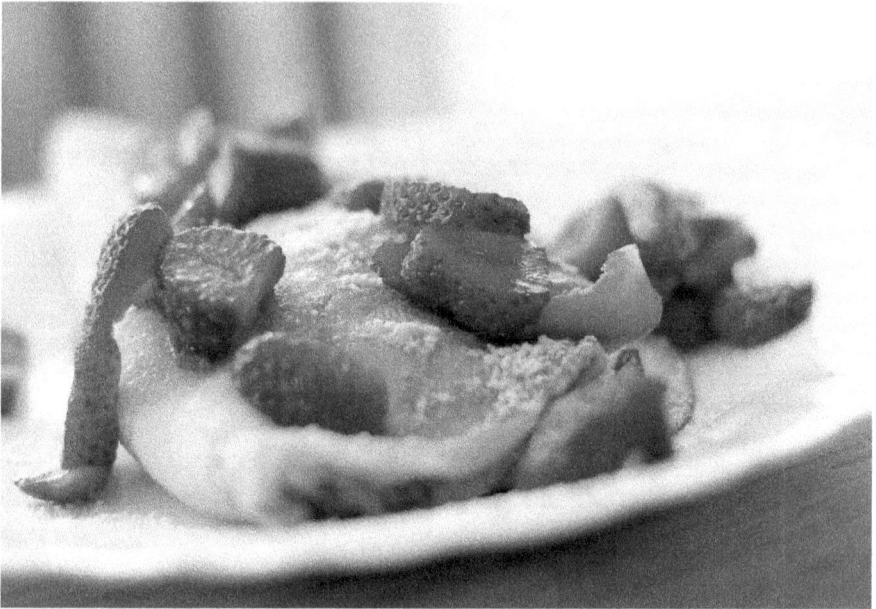

French Crepe

Servings Provided: 8

Time Required: 20 minutes

What is Needed:

The Crepes:

- Eggs (2)
- Melted butter (.25 cup)
- Sugar (2.5 tbsp.)

- A-P flour (.5 cup)
- Milk (.5 cup)
- Water (.125 cup)
- Vanilla (.5 tsp.)
- Dash (tiny dash)

  The Filling:

- Powdered sugar (2-4 tbsp./as desired)
- Heavy whipping cream (1 cup)
- Vanilla extract (.5 tsp.)
- Freshly sliced strawberries
- Also Needed: **Non-stick - 6-inch skillet**

Preparation Method:

1. Prepare the crepes. Whisk all the fixings except the flour.
2. Fold in the flour - a little bit at a time - whisking just until the flour is incorporated.
3. Let the crepe batter rest for ten minutes. Whisk again before using it.
4. Grease the skillet with unsalted butter and warm it using the medium-temperature setting.
5. Pour about two to three tablespoons of batter into the pan - while tipping the pan from side to side to get the mixture spreading over the pan.
6. Cook each side of the crepe for half a minute before gently loosening the edges with a large spatula. If it lifts, it's ready to be

flipped. If not, cook it for another 10-15 seconds and try again. Gently lift the crepe out of the pan, then flip over into the pan and cook the other side for another 10-15 seconds; remove to cool.

7. Prepare the filling. Use a hand/stand mixer to beat the heavy whipping cream until soft peaks form. Add in the powdered sugar and vanilla. Continue mixing until stiff peaks form.

8. Spread a layer of cream over each crepe, sliced strawberries, and roll the crepe as you would a wrap.

French Omelette

Servings Provided: 1

Time Required: 15 minutes

What is Needed:

- Milk (1 tbsp.)
- Egg (1)
- Basil (1 tbsp.)
- Chives (1 tbsp.)
- Tarragon (.5 tbsp.)
- Salt and pepper (a pinch of each)
- Olive oil (as needed for the pan)
- Sundried tomato (1 thinly sliced - oil drained)
- Crumbled goat cheese (1 tbsp.)

Preparation Method:

1. Chop the basil, tarragon, and chives.

2. Whisk the milk, egg, salt, and pepper in a small mixing container. Add half of the fresh herbs and gently stir to combine.

3. Add one tablespoon of olive oil to a small pan. Warm the oil using medium heat as you swirl it around the pan so that it coats the entire bottom of the pan and a little bit along the sides of the pan.

4. Dump the egg mixture into the pan. Swirl the pan so that the egg batter goes to the edges of the pan. Use a rubber spatula to gently push the egg batter to the edges of the pan.

5. Once the egg batter looks set on the bottom and is starting to bubble up a bit, lift the pan while tilting it to one side to slide the egg onto an awaiting using a large spatula. Flip the egg onto its other side into the pan and place it back on the burner using low heat.

6. Toss the crumbled cheese and tomato slices into the center of the omelet. Gently fold one side of the egg over, folding one more time - over itself (into thirds).

7. Serve promptly, garnished with the remaining fresh herbs.

Chapter 2: Delicious Salads

Traditional French Country Salad With Lemon Dijon
Vinaigrette

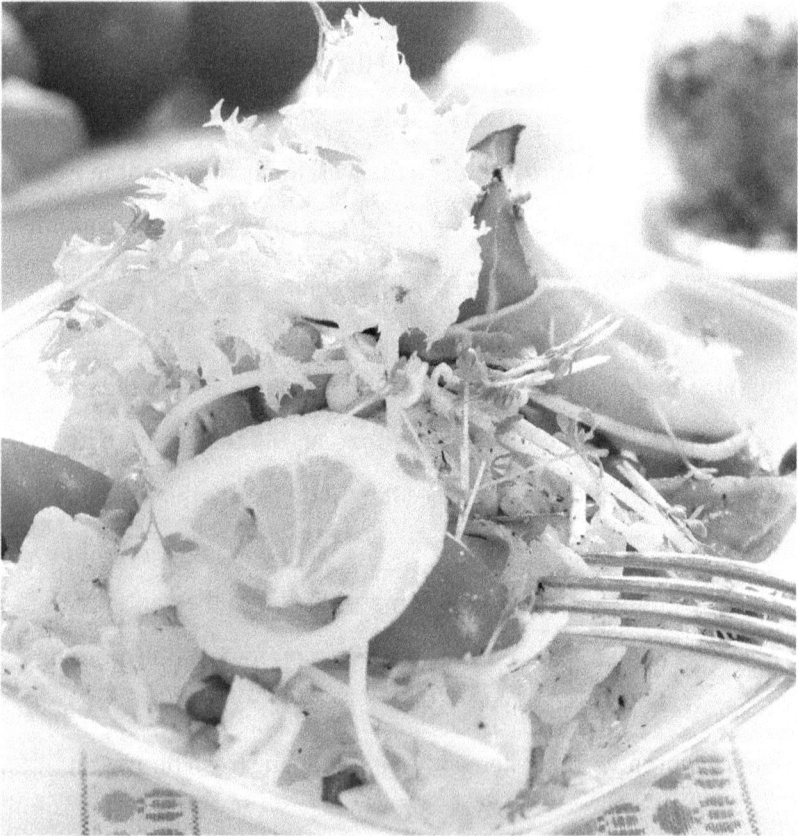

Servings Provided: 4

Time Required: 20 minutes

What is Needed:

- Arugula (5 oz. bag)
- Asparagus (.5 lb.)
- Olive oil (as desired)
- Sea salt (as desired)
- Sliced cooked beets (.5 cup)
- Whole walnuts or pecans, toasted (.5 cup)
- Crumbled goat cheese (.25 cup)
  The Vinaigrette:

- Balsamic vinegar (3 tbsp.)
- Dijon mustard (2 tbsp.)
- Olive oil (2 tbsp.)
- Minced garlic cloves (2 small)
- Sea salt & black pepper(.5 tsp./to taste)
- Lemon & zest (half of 1 lemon)

Preparation Method:

1. Set the oven at 400° Fahrenheit. Prepare a baking tray with a piece of parchment baking paper.

2. Trim the tattered ends and cut the asparagus into 1.5-inch long pieces. Spread it onto the prepared baking sheet. Drizzle the olive oil over the asparagus along with a sprinkle of sea salt.

3. Roast the asparagus for four to five minutes or until the asparagus is tender but still has a bite. Let it cool.

4. Toss the arugula with the asparagus in a large bowl.

5. Prepare the dressing. Whisk all of the vinaigrette fixings in a small measuring cup.

6. Assemble the salad. Toss the salad with the vinaigrette until

everything is lightly coated, and garnish it using sliced beets, toasted nuts, and crumbled goat cheese.

Chapter 3: Soup

Classic French Onion Bistro Soup

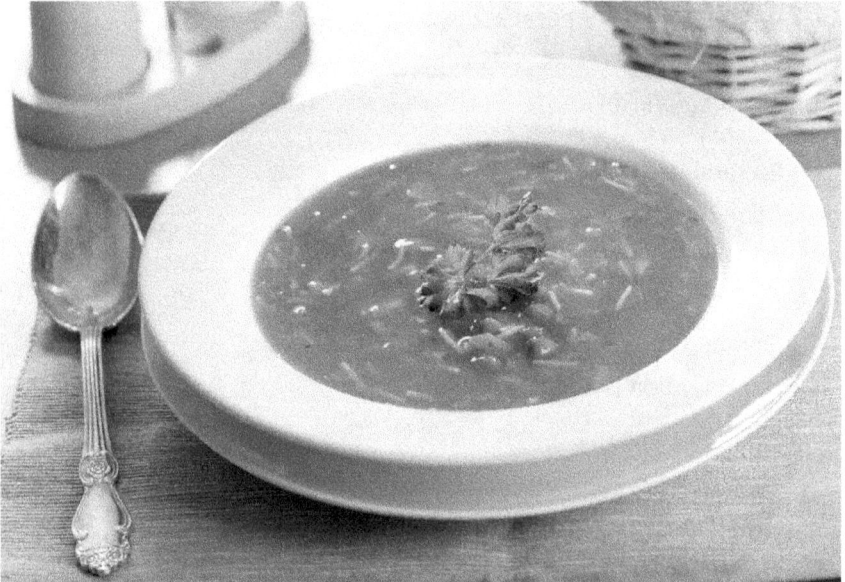

Servings Provided: 4

Time Required: 1.5 hours

What is Needed:

- Onions, (8 cups sliced/2 extra-large)
- Unsalted butter (1.5 tbsp.)
- Oil (1 tbsp.)
- Salt (.5 tsp.)
- Sugar (1 pinch)

- A-P flour (1.5 tbsp.)
- Low-sodium beef broth (4 cups)
- Pepper & salt (as desired)
- Sliced crusty French bread
- Gruyere cheese for the top/gruyere-cheddar mix (4 oz.)
- Also Needed: Oven-proof bowls (4)

Preparation Method:

1. Melt the butter with oil over low heat in a large pot or dutch oven. Slice the onions into crescent shapes and toss them into the pan. Place a lid on the pan and simmer them for about 15 minutes.
2. Slice the bread into ½-inch slices and toast them (set aside).
3. Adjust the stovetop temperature setting slightly higher and stir in the salt and sugar. Simmer with the lid off for another 40 to 45 minutes until onions have caramelized. Stir them occasionally throughout the duration.
4. Sprinkle the flour into the pot, stir, and simmer an additional three minutes.
5. Slowly add the broth into the pot, stirring as your pour. Season with a pinch of salt and pepper and cook for another 20 minutes until simmering and hot.
6. Warm the oven at 350° Fahrenheit.
7. Once the soup is ready, divide the soup into bowls. Place four to five baguette slices into each bowl. Top each bowl with grated cheese (.25 cup each dish).
8. Bake them until the cheese completely melts and serve promptly.

Fresh French Pea Soup

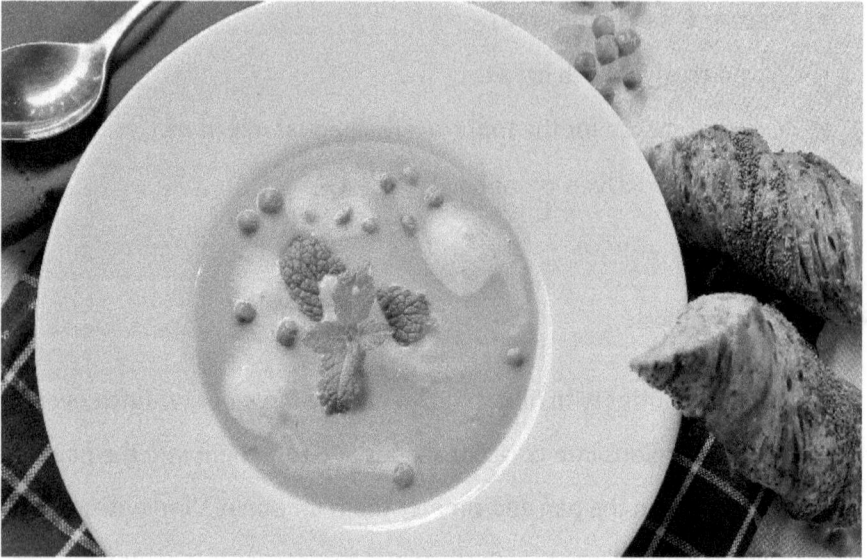

Servings Provided: 4

Time Required: 17 minutes

What is Needed:

- Butter with salt (2 tbsp.)
- Shallots (2 medium)
- Water (2 cups)
- Fresh green peas (3 cups)
- Table salt (.25 tsp.)
- Heavy whipping cream (3 tbsp.)

Preparation Method:

1. Prepare a heavy-bottomed saucepan (medium temp) to melt the butter. Sauté the shallots until soft and translucent (3 min.).
2. Pour in the water, peas, pepper, and salt. Adjust the temperature setting to med-high and bring to a boil.
3. Once boiling, lower the temperature setting to low, cover, and simmer until the peas are tender (12-18 min.).
4. Puree the peas in a food processor/blender in batches. Strain the pureed peas back into the saucepan, stir in the cream, and warm until it's piping hot.
5. Season to your liking with pepper and salt before serving.

Green Vegetable Soup

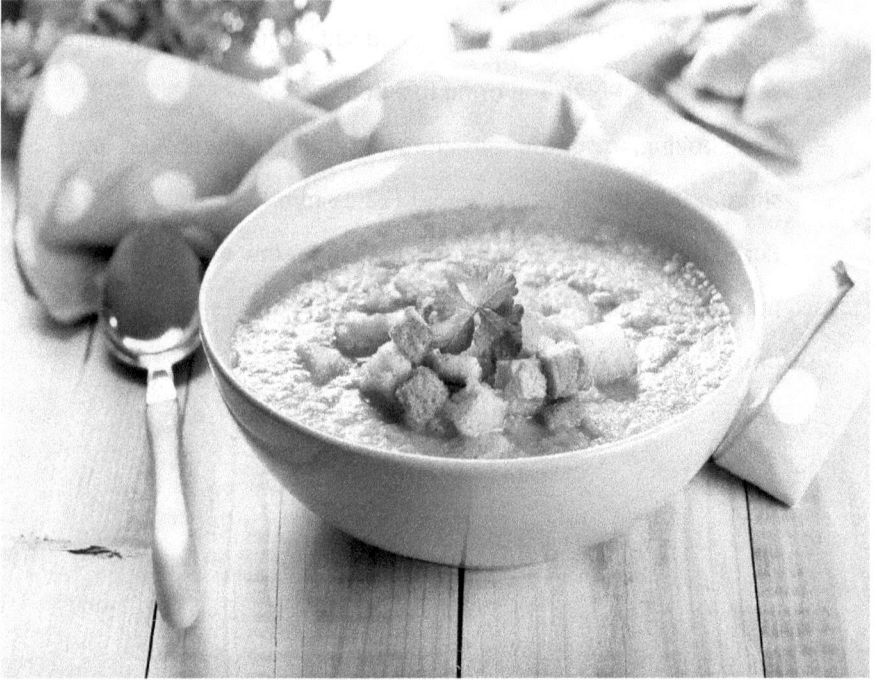

Servings Provided: 6

Time Required: 1 hour 40 minutes

What is Needed:

- Onions (2)
- Garlic (3 cloves)

- Butter, with salt (3 tbsp.)
- Swanson Clear Chicken Broth CAM (2 - 14.5 oz. cans)
- Water (4.5 cups)
- Carrots (3)
- Leeks (1)
- Spring onions/scallions - include tops & bulb (3)
- Habanero pepper (1 ½)
- Spinach (10 oz. bag)
- Watercress (1 bunch - raw)
- Table salt (1 tbsp.)
- Extra-virgin olive oil NOI (.25 cup)
- Red wine vinegar (50 Grain) NAK (.125 cup)

Preparation Method:

1. Warm a skillet using the med-high temperature setting. Sauté the minced garlic and onion (5 min.).
2. Add the water, chicken stock, spinach, carrots, green onions, leeks, habanero peppers, and watercress. Prepare it using a low-boil until the carrots are softened (30 min.). Remove the pan from the burner, and cool it for about half an hour.
3. When cooled, puree the soup in a food processor until smooth. Pour the mixture into the pot, and simmer using the low-temperature setting for 15 minutes.
4. Serve with a drizzle of olive oil and vinegar to your liking.

Chapter 4: Beef Options

Beef Bourguignon - Slow-Cooked

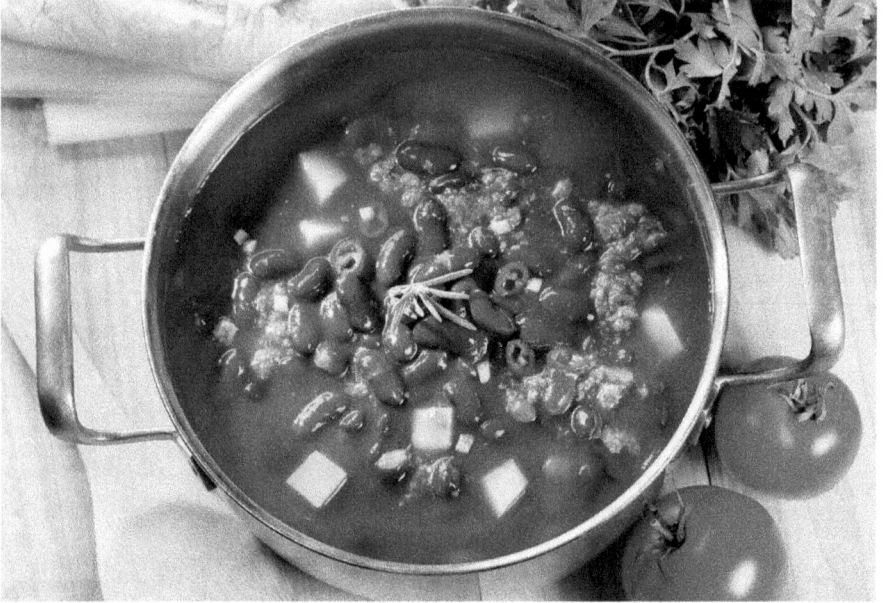

Servings Provided: 6

Time Required: 2.5 hours

What is Needed:

- Bacon (6 oz. - diced)
- Beef chuck (3 lb.)

- Large onion (1 chopped)
- Carrots (1)
- Garlic (2 minced cloves)
- A-P flour (3 tbsp.)
- Beef broth (1.5 cups)
- Red wine (¼ of a bottle)
- Salt (1 tsp.)
- Black pepper (1 pinch)
- Rosemary (1 sprig)
- Thyme (2 sprigs)
- Bay leaf (1)
- Olive oil (2 tbsp.)
- White mushrooms (7-8 thick slices)
- Pearl onions (10 oz.)
- For the Garnish: Fresh parsley

Preparation Method:

1. Warm a dutch oven or other large pot to cook the diced bacon using the med-high temperature setting. When it's nicely browned, transfer it to a paper-lined platter using a slotted spoon. Save the diced bacon for breakfast or a dish of mashed potatoes or just trash it.

2. Slice the beef into two-inch portions and toss it into the pot to brown each side. Remove the meat from the pan.

3. Chop and mix in the onion to sauté until it's translucent (5 min.).

Mince and add the garlic to sauté for about half a minute.

4. Add the beef back into the pot and dust it with three tablespoons of flour. Stir the meat until the flour has been absorbed (1 min.).

5. Add in the beef broth and just enough red wine to almost fully immerse it in juices. Stir and add a teaspoon of pepper and salt as desired.

6. Tie the rosemary, thyme, and bay leaf together with a piece of kitchen twine, and drop the bouquet into the pot. Slice the carrots in half lengthwise, then cut into one-inch wide pieces, and add the carrots into the pot as well. Simmer them using the medium temperature setting. Cover the pot with a lid and adjust the temperature setting to med-low. Simmer the stew for about 2.2 to 3 hours until the beef is very tender.

7. Warm the olive oil in a large skillet using the med-low temperature setting. Add the sliced mushrooms and pearl onions, cooking until both are softened (7-8 min.). Set aside until ready to serve.

8. After the beef is ready, remove the herb packet.

9. Prepare a shallow bowl with the meat, sautéed mushrooms, pearl onions, and carrots. Add the sauce and garnish with a portion of chopped parsley.

Entrecote Steak With Red Wine Sauce

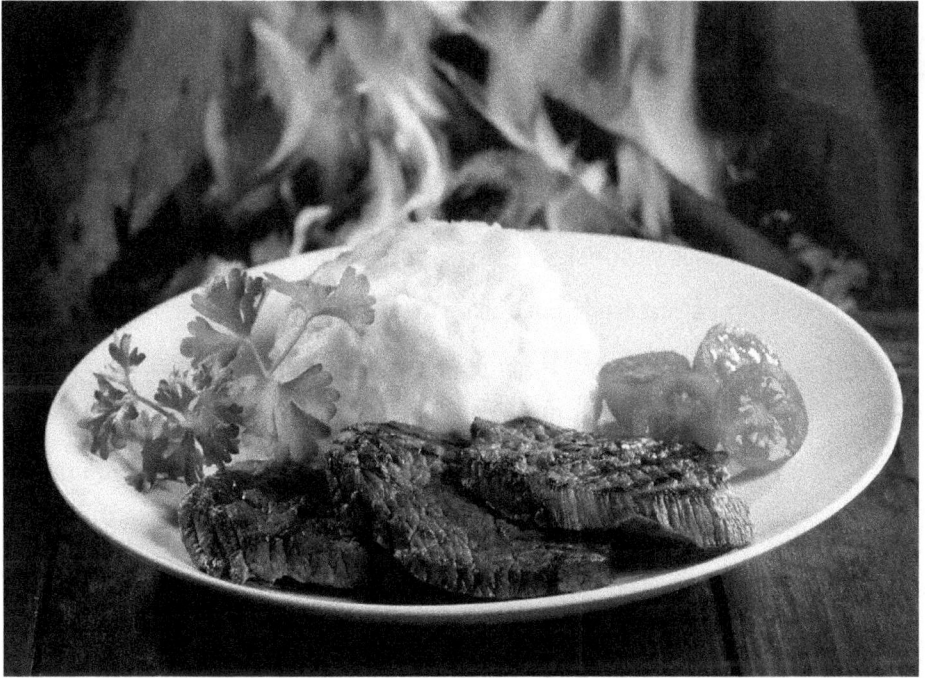

Servings Provided: 2

Time Required: 16 minutes

What is Needed:

- Rib-eye steaks (2 small)
- Black pepper & salt (as desired)
- Butter - unsalted (3 tbsp.)
- Shallot (1)

- Red wine (3 tbsp.)
- Beef stock (1/3 cup + 1 tbsp.)
- To Garnish: freshly chopped parsley

Preparation Method:

1. Generously sprinkle the steaks with pepper and salt.
2. Warm a cast-iron skillet using the high-temperature setting until it's 'smoking' hot. Add 1.5 tablespoons of butter to the pan, adjusting the setting to med-high.
3. Add the steaks to the hot buttered pan to cook for three minutes per side (medium doneness). Transfer the steaks to a platter for now.
4. Finely chop and add the shallot to the pan and sauté them for about a minute. Add the wine, and scrape the tasty browned bits with the juices from the bottom of the pan.
5. Reduce the temperature setting to medium, and stir in the beef stock. Simmer the mixture until the liquid has reduced by about half. Stir in the rest of the butter and prepare to serve it.
6. Use a sharp knife to slice the steaks at an angle and add the sauce. Garnish with a portion of fresh parsley.
7. Serve with your favorite side dish (ex. mashed potatoes, veggies, or french fries).

Pan-Seared Steak au Poivre

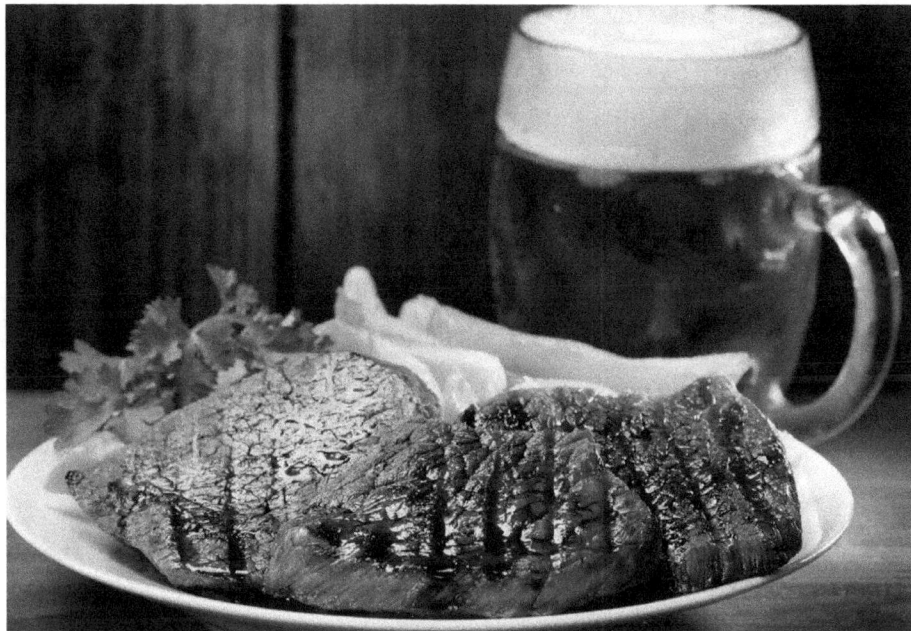

Servings Provided: 4

Time Required: 30 minutes

What is Needed:

- Filet mignons (4 small 1-inch each)
- Black peppercorns - cracked (1 tbsp.)
- Beef broth (.5 cup)
- Olive oil (1 tbsp.)
- Optional: Cognac (.25 cup)
- Cubed butter (2 tbsp.)

Preparation Method:

1. Use a paper towel to pat dry each filet and dust with pepper.
2. Warm a heavy cast-iron skillet using the medium-high heat until it's 'smoking' hot.
3. Flip the steaks and cook until small drops of red juice come to the surface (5 min. for medium). Transfer to a platter and keep them warm until time to add them to the mixture.
4. Empty the broth into the skillet to heat using the high-temperature setting and scrape up any browned bits.
5. At this point, add in the cognac and boil for one to two minutes to burn off the alcohol.
6. Remove the skillet from the burner. Whisk in the butter one cube at a time until melted.
7. Pour the sauce over the steaks and serve.

Steak Diane

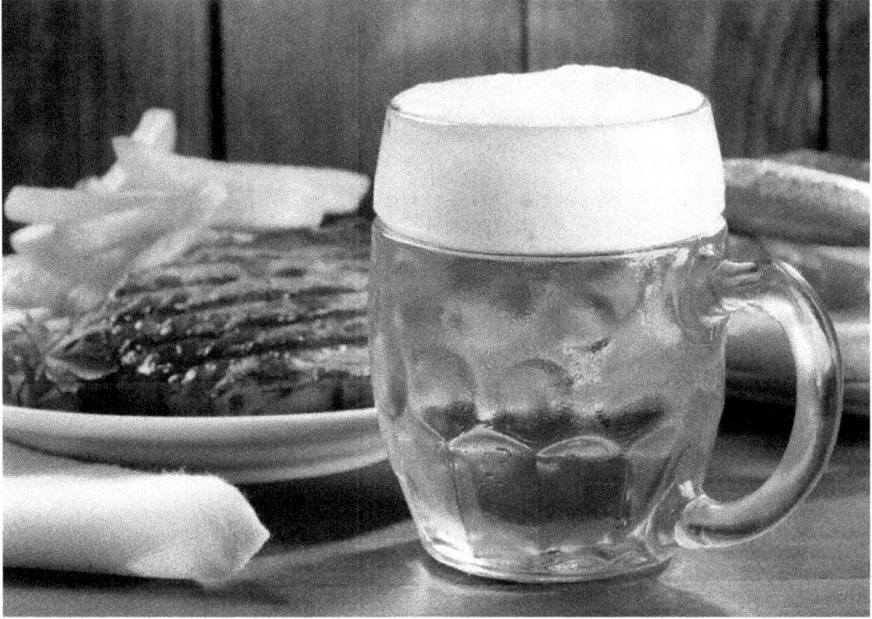

Servings Provided: 2

Time Required: 30 minutes

What is Needed:

- Jus De Veau Lie/Veal Demi-Glace-Pwd FD (.5 cup)
- Dijon Mustard NB (1 tbsp.)
- Worcestershire Sauce (2 tsp.)
- Tomato paste - salt added (1 tsp. - canned)
- Spices - pepper, red or cayenne (1 pinch)
  The Steaks:

- Soybean oil (2 tsp.)
- Beef tenderloin (2 - 8 oz. trimmed to ¼- inch thickness)
- Black pepper & kosher salt (as desired)
- Butter - no-salt (1 tbsp.)
- Shallots (3 tbsp.)

- Cognac (.25 cup)
- Heavy whipping cream (.25 cup)
- Chives (2 tsp.)

Preparation Method:

1. Generously sprinkle the steaks with salt. Wait for them to reach room temperature while you make the sauce.

2. Use the high-temperature setting to warm the oil. Once it reaches a smoking point, add the steaks, and dot them with a few chunks of butter.

3. Sear the meat (high temp) until brown on each side, two to three minutes on each side, keeping them on the rare side (internal temp of 125° Fahrenheit. Transfer steaks to a warm plate.

4. Toss the shallots into the skillet and sauté them until softened (2-3 min.).

5. Remove the skillet to a cool burner and add in the Cognac. Carefully ignite it using a fireplace lighter. After the alcohol burns off and the flames go out, return the skillet to the high setting and wait for it to boil. Simmer for a few minutes to reduce its volume slightly.

6. Add demi-glace mixture, cream, and any accumulated juices from the steak. Cook on high heat just until the sauce starts to thicken (3-5 min.).

7. Transfer the steaks back into the pan and adjust the temperature setting to low. Gently simmer until meat is heated through and cooked to your desired level of doneness.

8. Serve on a heated plate with a generous portion of sauce. Sprinkle with chives to your liking and serve.

Chapter 5: Other Delicious French Classics

French Ham & Grilled Cheese Sandwich - Croque Monsieur

Servings Provided: 4

Time Required: 25 minutes

What is Needed:

- Sourdough toast (8 slices)
- Gruyere cheese (8 oz.)
- Black forest ham (8 slices)
- Bechamel sauce (1 recipe)
- Dijon mustard

  The Sauce:

- Whole milk (1 cup)
- Unsalted butter (1 tbsp.)
- A-P flour (2 tbsp.)
- Pepper and salt (to your liking)

Preparation Method:

1. Make the sauce by warming the milk in a small saucepan using the med-low temperature setting until steam rises from the milk, but it has yet to boil. *Don't boil.*

2. Use another saucepan to melt the butter. Sift in the flour to create a bubbly, paste-like mixture. Slowly pour in hot milk, whisking it with a pinch of salt and pepper to your liking.

3. Stir the bechamel sauce using the low-temperature setting until it's thick enough to coat the back of a wooden spoon.

4. Set the oven using the broil function. Toast the bread slices and spread them with the mustard over half of the bread.

5. Prepare the sandwich using two slices of ham and shredded cheese on each. Top it using the ham with more shredded cheese.

6. Put the remaining bread slices over the ham and cheese to assemble the sandwiches. Spread about one to two tablespoons of bechamel sauce over the top of each sandwich. Sprinkle more shredded cheese on top of the bechamel.

7. Place the sandwiches on a baking tray and place the pan on the center oven rack until the cheese starts to melt.

8. Move the sandwiches to the top rack for about 30 seconds, removing when the cheese starts to obtain little golden spots.

Pork Chops With Mustard Sauce

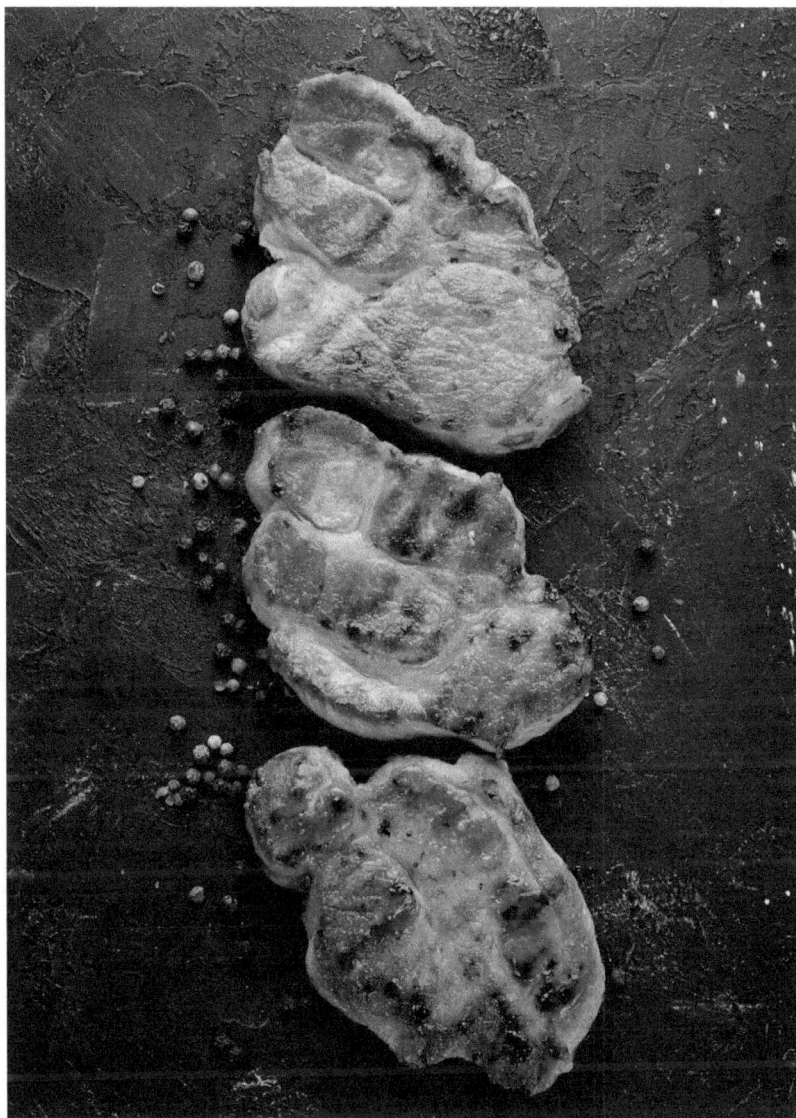

Servings Provided: 4

Time Required: 20 minutes

What is Needed:

- Olive oil (3 tbsp.)
- Boneless pork chops (4 - 1-inch or 1.5 lb.)
- Black pepper & kosher salt (.5 tsp. each/as desired)
- Finely chopped shallots (2)
- Dry white wine (.75 cup)
- Heavy cream (2 tbsp.)
- Dijon mustard (1 tbsp.)
- Freshly chopped tarragon (1 tbsp.)
- Torn frisée pieces (1 small head/4 cups)
- Lemon wedges (1)

Preparation Method:

1. Heat oven to 400° Fahrenheit.

2. Warm one tablespoon of the oil in a large skillet using the medium-high temperature setting.

3. Sprinkle the pork using pepper and salt. Let them cook and brown for two to three minutes per side.

4. Transfer the pork to a baking tray and roast until thoroughly cooked (5-7 min.).

5. Meanwhile, add the shallots and one tablespoon of the oil to the skillet and cook, often stirring, until softened (3-4 min.)

6. Add the wine to the skillet and simmer until reduced by half. Add the cream and simmer until the sauce just thickens. Stir in the mustard.

7. Top the pork with the sauce and tarragon. Drizzle the frisée with the remaining tablespoon of oil and serve with the lemon wedges.

Provencal Chicken Casserole

Servings Provided: 4

Time Required: 53 minutes

What is Needed:

- Olive oil (5 tbsp.)
- Chicken - broilers/fryers/breast - meat only (4 @ 6 oz.)
- Lemon juice (1 lemon)
- Table salt (1 pinch)
- Cherry tomatoes (1.5 cups)
- Onions - Spring/scallions - include tops & bulb (1 bunch)
- Swanson Clear Chicken Broth CAM (.5 cup)
- Brown mustard - prepared (2 tbsp.)
- Fresh rosemary (1.5 sprigs)
- Fresh thyme (half bunch)
- Cheese - gruyere (2 cups)

Preparation Method:

1. Pour three tablespoons of olive oil into a shallow platter and lay chicken breasts on top. Rub with lemon juice, salt, and pepper.
2. Warm two tablespoons of olive oil in a nonstick skillet using the med-high temperature function. Cook the chicken breasts until browned (4 min. per side).

3. Preheat the oven at 350° Fahrenheit. Grease a baking dish. Place tomatoes and green onions in the baking dish and pour the chicken broth on top.

4. Whisk the mustard, rosemary, and thyme in a small bowl and brush onto chicken breasts. Arrange the chicken breasts on top of the vegetables in the baking dish. Cover with the Gruyere cheese.

5. Bake the casserole on the middle rack until the chicken juices run clear and are no longer pink in the center (30 min.). (You can test it using an instant-read thermometer inserted into the center for a reading of at least 165° Fahrenheit.)

White Wine Coq Au Vin

Servings Provided: 6

Time Required: 55 minutes

What is Needed:

- Chicken - thighs, breasts & drumsticks (8 pieces/3 lb.)
- Black pepper & kosher salt
- Unsalted butter (2 tbsp.)
- Sliced bacon (4 diced)
- Large sweet onion (1)
- Garlic (3 minced cloves)
- Cremini mushrooms (1 pint - sliced)

- Dry white wine (2 cups)
- Whole-grain mustard (1 tbsp.)
- Heavy cream (.5 cup)
- Freshly chopped parsley (.25 cup)

Preparation Method:

1. Season the chicken with pepper and salt. Melt the butter in a large skillet using the medium temperature setting.
2. Arrange the chicken in the skillet and cook until it's well browned (4 min. per side).
3. Transfer the chicken from the skillet and set it aside. Add the bacon to the skillet and cook until the fat begins to render (3 min.).
4. Dice and mix in the onion and sauté until it is translucent (5 min.). Add the garlic and mushrooms, and sauté until the mushrooms are tender (5-6 min.).
5. Add the browned chicken back to the skillet. Pour the wine into the skillet, stir in the mustard, and bring the mixture to a simmer using the med-low temperature function. Cover the skillet and simmer until the chicken is almost fully cooked (15-20 min.).
6. Uncover the skillet and add the cream. Simmer until the sauce thickens and the chicken is fully cooked (8-10 min.).
7. Garnish with parsley and serve immediately.

PART V

Chapter 1: Soup

Hot & Sour Soup

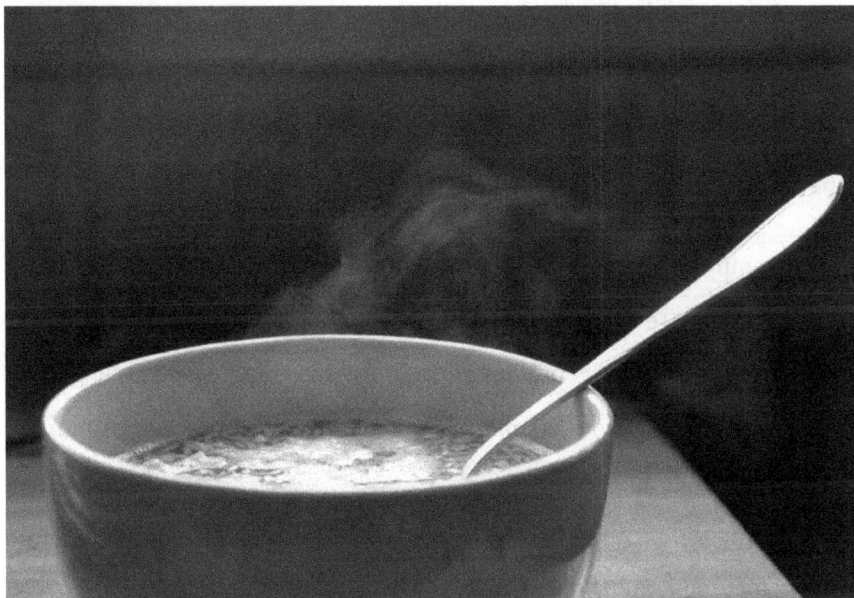

Servings Provided: 4

Time Required: 40 minutes

What is Needed:

- Chicken broth - low-sodium (1 quart)
- Dried tree ear fungus (.25 cup)
- Dried lily buds (12)
- Medium-dark soy sauce (2 tbsp. + more for seasoning)
- Distilled white vinegar (2 tbsp. + more for seasoning)
- Cornstarch (2 tbsp.)
- Kosher salt (.5 tsp.)
- Large eggs (2)

- Bamboo shoots (.5 cup - shredded)
- Cooked pork, ham, or chicken (.5 cup - shredded)
- Spiced thick - dry tofu - shredded (1 cup/3.5 oz.)
- White pepper - finely ground (1.5 tsp.)
- Sesame oil (1 tbsp.)
- To serve: Chopped cilantro & scallions

Preparation Method:

1. Dump the lily buds into boiling water to soak about ten minutes until they're softened. Discard the rough tips.

2. Prepare another container and add the tree fungus and boiling water to soak from 20 minutes to half an hour. Rinse, drain, and coarsely chop them.

3. Dump the broth into a large saucepan. Once boiling, add the soy sauce, salt, and vinegar.

4. Whisk three tablespoons of water with the cornstarch and mix it into the broth to simmer for three to four minutes to thicken.

5. Once it's at a rolling boil, whisk the eggs and a dash of salt, and work it into the soup in a circular fashion. Wait five seconds, stir and extinguish the heat.

6. Toss in the tofu, chicken, white pepper, bamboo shoots, ear fungus, and lily buds.

7. Simmer the soup using the medium temperature setting for about two minutes, adding in vinegar, soy sauce, and salt as desired.

8. Portion the soup and garnish it using the cilantro, scallions, and a spritz of sesame oil.

Wonton Soup

Servings Provided: 8

Time Required: 1 hour 15 minutes

What is Needed:

- Pork - fresh loin - whole (.5 lb.)
- Crustaceans - shrimp - mixed-species - raw (2 oz.)
- Brown sugar (1 tsp.)
- Burgundy wine (1 tbsp.)
- Shoyu - low-sodium soy sauce (1 tbsp.)
- Spring onions/scallions - tops & bulb (1 tsp.)
- Ginger root (1 tsp.)
- Wonton wrappers - includes egg roll wrappers (24 @ 3.5-inch square)
- Clear chicken broth - Swanson - CAM (3 cups)
- Scallions (includes tops and bulb- (1/8 cup)

Preparation Method:

1. Chop the green onion and add one teaspoon into a large mixing container and add the pork, shrimp, sugar, wine, shoyu sauce, and ginger. Thoroughly toss the mixture and let stand for 25 to 30 minutes.
2. Scoop the filling (1 tsp.) into the middle of each wonton skin.

3. Moisten the four edges of the wonton wrapper with a small amount of water on your fingertips, and pull the top corner down to the bottom, folding the wrapper over the filling to create a triangle.

4. Seal it by pressing the edges firmly. Bring the left and right corners together above the filling and overlap the corner of the tips. Moisten with water and press together. Repeat the process until all wrappers are used.

5. Make the soup. Heat the chicken stock to a rolling boil. Add the wontons and cook for five minutes.

6. Top off the soup with chopped green onions and serve.

Chapter 2: Seafood

Honey Walnut Shrimp

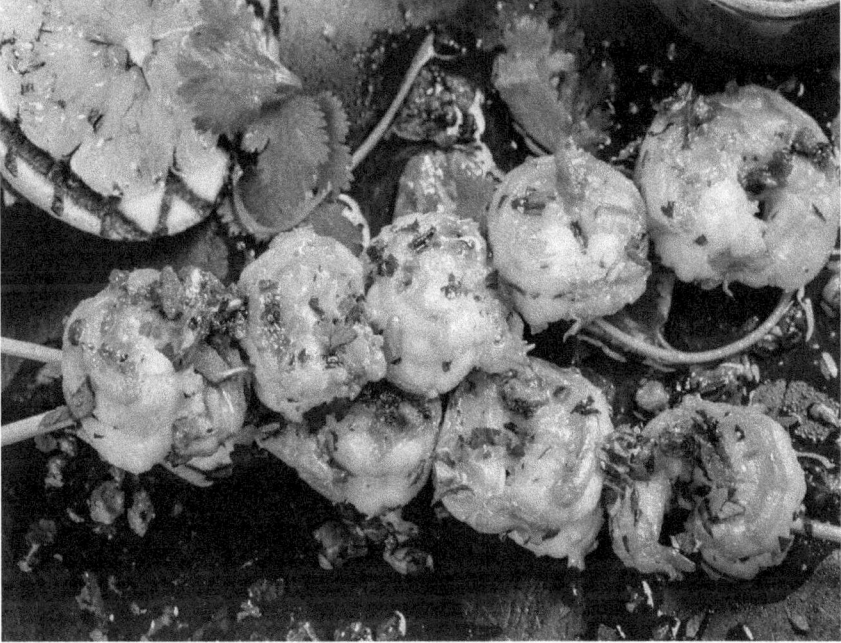

Servings Provided: 4

Time Required: 30 minutes

What is Needed:

- Water (1 cup)
- English walnuts (.5 cup)
- Granulated sugar (2/3 cup)

- Egg white - raw (4)
- Rice flour - white (2/3 cup)
- Salad dressing/soybean oil with salt/mayonnaise (.25 cup)
- Jumbo shrimp - fresh & raw (1 lb./21-30)
- Honey - strained or extracted (2 tbsp.)
- Sweet condensed canned milk (1 tbsp.)
- Oil for frying (1 cup)

Preparation Method:

1. Whisk the water and sugar in a small saucepan. Once boiling, add the walnuts and boil them for two minutes. Dump them into a colander to drain. Arrange the nuts on a baking tray to thoroughly dry.
2. Whip the egg whites in a mixing container until they're foamy. Stir in the mochiko until it's a pasty consistency.
3. Warm the oil using the med-high temperature setting in a heavy deep skillet.
4. Dip the shrimp into the batter, and fry them until nicely browned (5 min.). Transfer them to a paper towel-lined platter using a slotted spoon to allow them to drain.
5. Whisk the honey, mayonnaise, and sweetened condensed milk. Fold in the shrimp and toss to coat with the sauce.
6. Garnish using the candied walnuts right before serving.

Steamed Fish

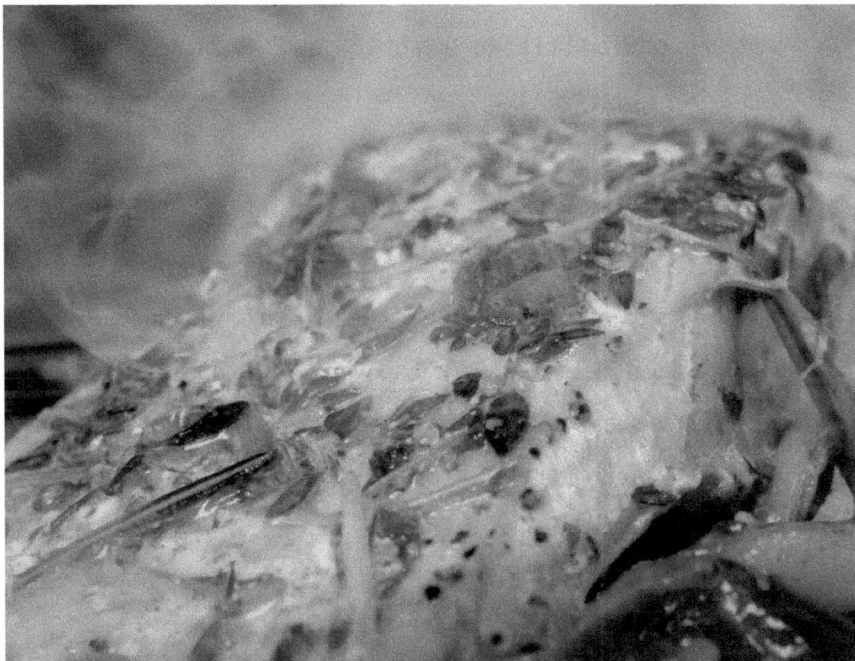

Servings Provided: 2

Time Required: 35 minutes

What is Needed:

- Raw finfish, snapper, mixed species (1 lb.)
- Salt (.5 tsp.)
- Black pepper (.5 tsp.)
- Ginger root - raw (1 tbsp.)
- Shoyu soy sauce (1 tbsp.)
- Sesame oil (2 tsp.)

- Shiitake mushrooms - raw AMM (2)
- Tomatoes (1 fresh)
- Peppers - raw red-hot chile (half of 1)
- Cilantro (2 sprigs - raw)

Preparation Method:

1. Prepare a steamer with a basket large enough for the snapper to lie flat. Pour in 1.5 inches of water and wait for it to boil.

2. Sprinkle the snapper with pepper and salt and pepper before placing it into the basket. Top the fish with ginger, and drizzle with sesame oil and soy sauce.

3. Place the tomatoes, mushrooms, and red chile pepper in the steamer basket.

4. Set a timer and steam the fish for 15 minutes, or until easily flaked with a fork. Garnish with cilantro and serve.

Stir-Fried Shrimp & Scallions

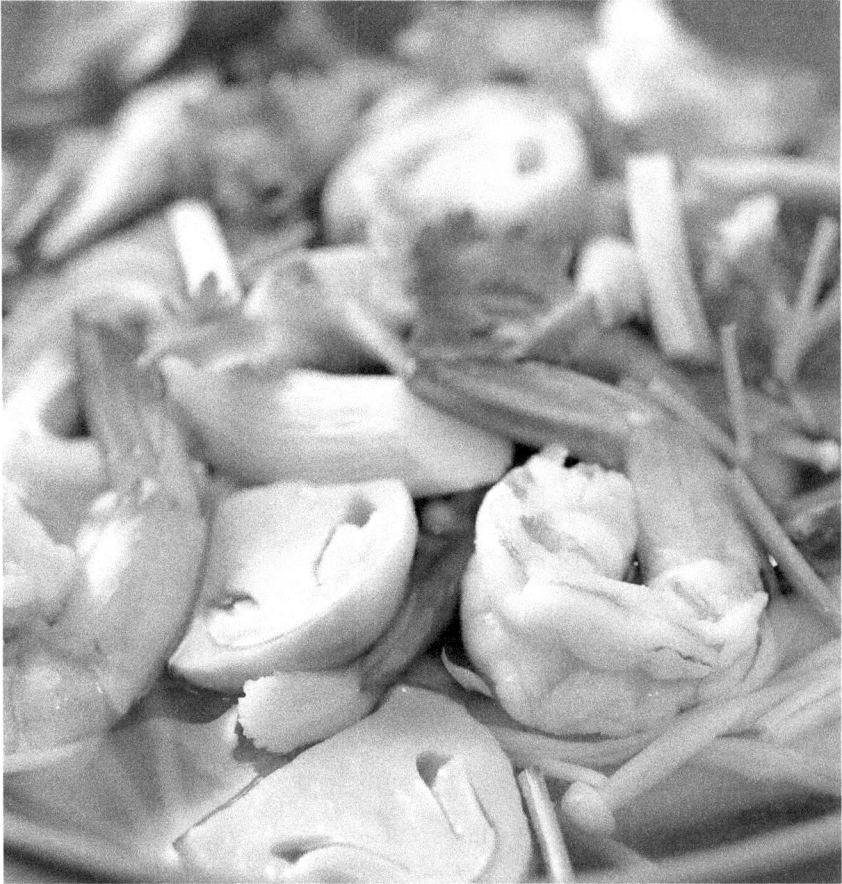

Servings Provided: 4

Time Required: 30 minutes

What is Needed:

- Jumbo shrimp (1.5 lb.)

- Garlic (3 cloves)
- Fresh ginger (1-inch section)
- Crushed red pepper (1.5 tsp.)
- Egg white (1 large)
- Cornstarch (2 tsp. - divided)
- Ketchup (.75 cup)
- Chicken broth - low-sodium (.5 cup)
- Black pepper & kosher salt (1.5 tsp. each)
- Sugar (1 tbsp.)
- Canola oil (.25 cup)
- Chopped cilantro (.5 cup)
- Scallions (3)

Preparation Method:

1. Thinly slice the scallions. Shell and devein the shrimp. Mince the garlic and ginger.
2. Toss the shrimp with the ginger, garlic, red pepper, one teaspoon of the cornstarch, and egg white until well-coated.
3. Whisk the broth with the ketchup, sugar, salt, and pepper with the rest of the cornstarch.
4. Warm a large skillet with the oil until it shimmers. Add the shrimp and stir-fry using the high-temperature setting until pink.
5. Add the ketchup mixture and simmer until the shrimp are heated (2 min.). Stir in the cilantro and scallions to serve.

Chapter 3: Poultry

Kung Pao Chicken - Keto-Friendly

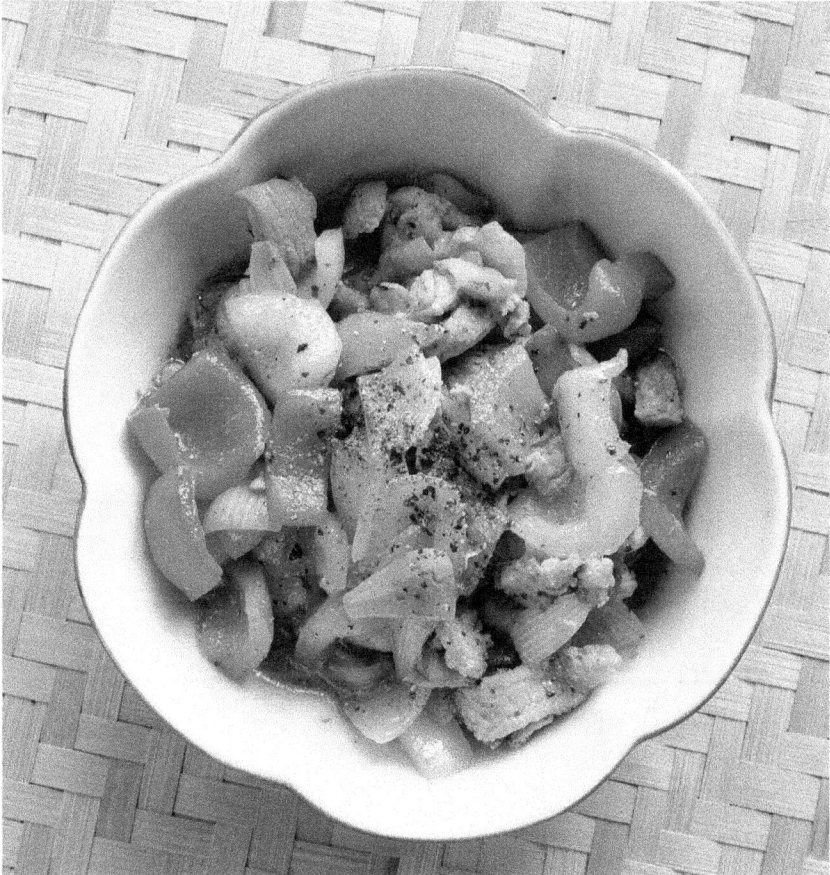

Servings Provided: 4

Time Required: 40 minutes

What is Needed:

- Chicken breasts - boneless skinless (1 lb.)

The Marinade:

- Chinese rice wine/dry sherry (2 tsp.)
- Soy sauce (2 tsp.)
- Cornstarch (2 tsp.)

To Cook:

- Olive oil or sunflower oil (3 tbsp. divided)
- Dried red chilies (4-6)
- Green onions (4)
- Optional: Red finger chili (1)
- Asparagus (1 bunch)
- Sweet bell pepper (1)
- Garlic & ginger (4 tsp. each)
- Mini cucumbers (2)
- Roasted salted peanuts/cashews (.33 cup)
- Toasted sesame seeds (1 tsp.)

The Sauce:

- Water (3 tbsp. - cold)
- Soy sauce & white vinegar (2 tbsp. each)
- Chinese wine/ sherry (1 tbsp.)
- Cornstarch (2 tsp.)
- Salt (.5 tsp.)
- Optional: Asian chili-garlic sauce (1 tbsp.)

Preparation Method:

1. Slice the chicken into one-inch chunks and combine it with the marinade fixings in the first group (soy sauce, rice wine, and cornstarch) stirring to combine. Marinate the mixture for 15

minutes.

2. Prep the veggies by cutting the asparagus into large pieces and mincing the garlic and onion. Chop the cucumber. Core and cube the bell pepper. Cut the green onions into one-inch pieces.

3. Prepare a large-sized cast-iron pan to warm one tablespoon of oil using the med-high temperature setting. Add the green onions, dried chilies, and finger chili.

4. Simmer the mixture until the green onions are slightly charred (1 min.). Transfer them to a baking sheet or large platter.

5. Heat the rest of the oil in the pan (1 tbsp.). Add asparagus and bell pepper and cook, stirring until it's slightly charred (2-3 min.).

6. Transfer to a baking tray and add the remainder of the oil (1.5 tsp.) to the pan. Working in two batches, stir-fry the chicken until browned (3-4 min. per batch), repeating with remaining oil.

7. Make the Sauce: Whisk the water, rice wine, soy sauce, and cornstarch until smooth. Return the chicken, vegetables, and chilies to the pan.

8. Sprinkle with salt, stir in the sauce, and cook until the liquid is bubbling and thickened (30 seconds to one minute). Stir in the cucumbers, peanuts, and chili-garlic sauce.

9. Serve it with a garnish of sesame seeds.

Orange Chicken

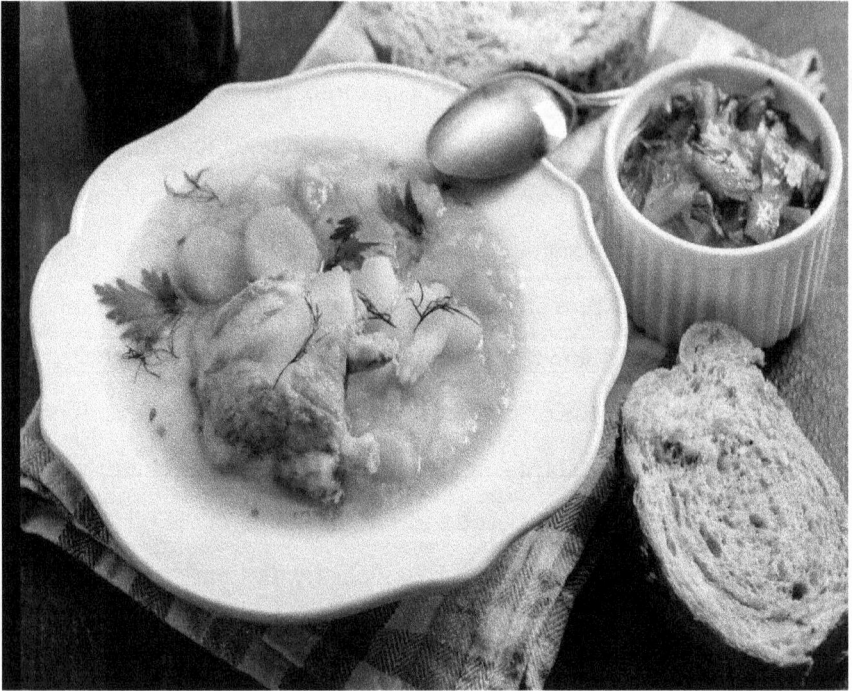

Servings Provided: 4

Time Required: 35 minutes

What is Needed:

The Chicken:

- Oil (as needed for frying)
- Boneless & skinless chicken breasts (4)
- Eggs (3 whisked)
- Cornstarch (.33 cup)

- Flour (.33 cup)

  Orange Chicken Sauce:

- Orange juice (1 cup)
- Sugar (.5 cup)
- Rice/white vinegar (2 tbsp.)
- Tamari or soy sauce (2 tbsp.)
- Ginger (.25 tsp.)
- Garlic powder (.25 tsp.) or 2 garlic cloves (2 finely diced)
- Red chili flakes (.5 tsp.)
- Orange Zest (1 orange)
- Cornstarch (1 tbsp.)

  The Garnish:

- Orange Zest
- Green Onions

Preparation Method:

1. Prepare the orange sauce. Mince the ginger and garlic. Pour the vinegar, orange juice, soy sauce, sugar, garlic, ginger, and red chili flakes into a saucepan. Sauté them for about three minutes.

2. Whisk one tablespoon of cornstarch with two tablespoons of water to form a paste. Add it to the orange sauce and whisk thoroughly. Continue cooking the sauce for about five minutes, until the mixture begins to thicken. After it's thickened, remove the pan from the burner and add the orange zest.

3. Prepare the chicken by cutting it into bite-sized chunks.

4. Dump the flour, a pinch of salt, and cornstarch in a pie plate or another shallow dish.

5. Whisk eggs in a shallow mixing container.

6. Dip the pieces of chicken into the egg mix and then flour mixture. Place them onto a platter.

7. Next, warm two to three inches of oil in a heavy-bottomed skillet (med-high temperature). Use an electric skillet or use a thermometer to check the heat until it reaches 350° Fahrenheit.

8. Working in batches, fry several chicken pieces at a time. Cook them for two to three minutes, often turning until golden brown, and place the chicken on a paper-towel-lined plate. Repeat the process until all the chicken is cooked.

9. Toss the chicken with the orange sauce. Reserve some of the sauce to serve over the rice. Serve it with a sprinkling of green onion and orange zest to your liking.

Chapter 4: Pork

Chinese Pork BBQ (Char Siu)

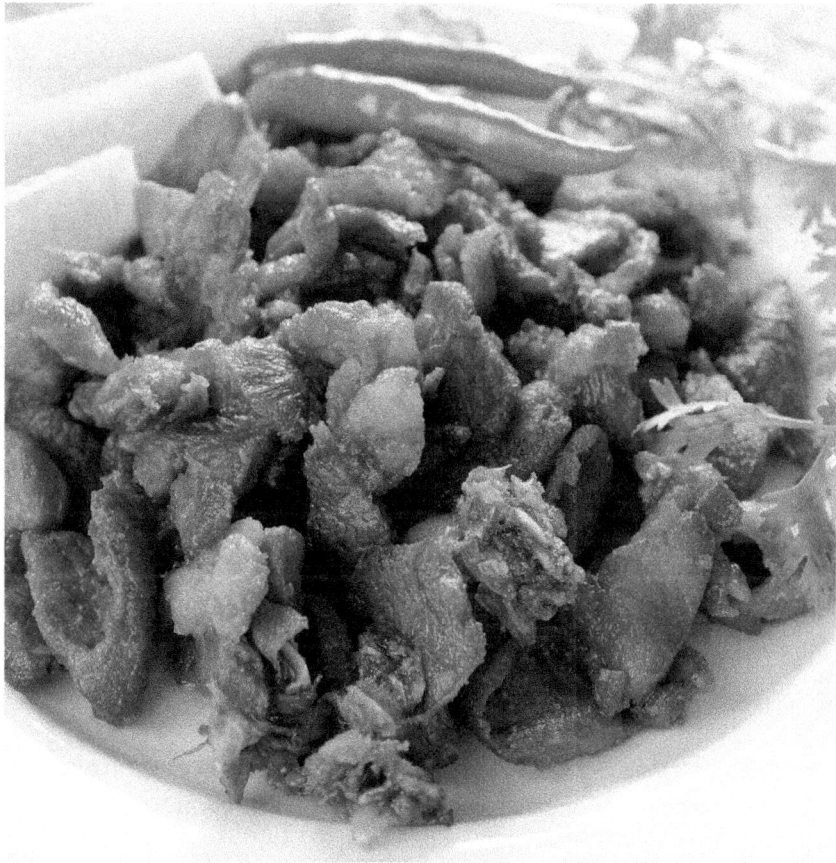

Servings Provided: 4

Time Required: 3 hours 40 minutes

What is Needed:

- Fresh pork tenderloin - lean cut (2 lb.)
- Soy sauce -shoyu - made from soy and wheat (.5 cup)
- Honey - strained/extracted (.33 cup)
- Ketchup (.33 cup)
- Brown sugar (.33 cup)
- Hoisin sauce - ready-to-serve (2 tbsp.)
- Rice wine (.25 cup)
- Red food coloring (.5 tsp.)
- Chinese Five-Spice Powder (1 tsp.)

Preparation Method:

1. Cut the pork "with the grain" into strips 1.5-2-inches long, and toss it into a large resealable zipper-type baggie.

2. Whisk the soy sauce, ketchup, honey, hoisin sauce, brown sugar, red food coloring, Chinese 5-spice, and rice wine in a saucepan using the med-low temperature setting. Simmer it until just combined and slightly warm (2-3 min.). Pour the marinade into the bag with the pork, pushing the air from the bag, and zip it closed. Toss the bag several times to cover all pork pieces.

3. Pop the pork in the fridge for two hours or overnight.

4. Warm the outdoor grill using the med-high temperature setting and lightly grease the grate.

5. Transfer the pork from marinade, shaking it to remove excess juices. Discard the marinade.

6. Grill the pork for 20 minutes. Place a container of water onto the grill and continue cooking, turning the pork until cooked thoroughly or about one hour. It's ready when the internal temp reaches 145°

Fahrenheit.

Chinese Pork Dumplings

Servings Provided: 5/50 dumplings

Time Required: 1 hour 20 minutes

What is Needed:

- Soy sauce made from wheat & soy - shoyu (.5 cup)
- White rice vinegar CBT (1 tbsp.)
- Chinese chive - kucai - raw (1 tbsp.)
- Dried sesame seeds - whole (1 tbsp.)
- Sriracha sauce/Chili puree sauce w/Garlic CBT (1 tsp.)
- Freshly ground pork - raw (1 lb.)
- Garlic (3 cloves)
- Egg - whole (1)
- Kucai - Chinese chive - raw (2 tbsp.)

Preparation Method:

1. Combine ½ cup of the soy sauce, rice vinegar, sesame seeds, one tablespoon of chives, and the chile sauce in a small mixing container. Set it to the side for now.

2. Mix the pork, minced garlic, egg, two tablespoons of chives, soy sauce, sesame oil, and ginger in a large mixing container until thoroughly combined.

3. Lightly flour a workspace. Place a dumpling wrapper onto it and spoon about one tablespoon of the filling in the center.

4. Wet the edge with a little water and crimp it together, forming small pleats to seal the dumpling. Repeat the process with the rest of the dumpling wrappers and filling.

5. Warm one to two tablespoons of oil in a large skillet using the med-high temperature setting. Arrange eight to ten dumplings in the pan and cook until browned (2 min. per side).

6. Pour in one cup of water, place a lid on the pot, and simmer until the pork is thoroughly cooked and the dumplings are tender (5 min.).

7. Continue the process until all dumplings are prepared. Serve with the soy sauce mixture for dipping.

Chop Suey

Servings Provided: 6

Time Required: 51 minutes

What is Needed:

- Fresh pork tenderloin (1 lb.)
- Wheat flour, all-purpose, white, enriched, bleached (.25 cup)
- Oil - soybean, salad or cooking (2 tbsp.)
- Bok choy - raw (2 cups)
- Celery - fresh (1 cup)
- Sweet red bell peppers (1 cup)
- Mushrooms (1 cup)
- Water chestnuts, Chinese, canned - solids & liquids (8 oz. can)
- Garlic (2 fresh cloves)
- Swanson Clear Chicken Broth CAM (.25 cup)
- Shoyu sauce (.25 cup)
- Cornstarch (1 tbsp.)
- Fleischmann's Cooking Sherry II (1 tbsp.)
- Ground ginger (.5 tsp.)

Preparation Method:

1. Use a sharp knife to discard the fat from the pork and slice it into one-inch pieces. Combine the flour and pork in a resealable bag, seal, and shake it thoroughly to cover.

2. Warm one tablespoon oil in a large skillet using the med-high heat setting. Add the trimmed pork and cook for three minutes or until browned. Transfer it to a container and keep it warm.

3. Pour the rest of the oil in the pan to heat. Add the celery, bok choy, mushrooms, red pepper, garlic, and water chestnuts. Stir-fry them for three minutes.

4. Thoroughly whisk the chicken broth, soy sauce, cornstarch, sherry, and ginger in a mixing container.

5. Combine the pork and broth mixture in a skillet, and cook for one minute or until thickened.

Easy Moo Shu Pork

Servings Provided: 6

Time Required: 1 hour 20 minutes

What is Needed:

- *Shoyu* - Soy sauce made from soy + wheat (2 tbsp.)
- Sesame oil (1 tbsp.)
- Garlic (1 tsp.)
- Fresh ginger root (1 tbsp.)
- Pork tenderloin (.75 lb.)
- Oil - soybean - salad or cooking (2 tbsp.)
- Chinese cabbage (pe-tsai) (2 cups)
- Carrots (1 raw)
- Salt (1 pinch)

Preparation Method:

1. Whisk the sesame oil, soy sauce, garlic and ginger in a bowl until the marinade is smooth. Dump it into a resealable plastic bag and add the pork. Cover it using the marinade, squeeze out any excess air, and seal the bag. Marinate in the fridge for a minimum of one hour to overnight.

2. Warm vegetable oil in a wok/large skillet using the medium temperature setting. Rinse and add the cabbage and diced carrot. Simmer the mixture for one to two minutes.

3. Push the cabbage mixture aside and add pork with marinade to the center of the skillet. Cook and stir until the pork is thoroughly cooked (3-4 min.).

4. Scoot the cabbage into the center of the skillet and continue to cook it for another minute or two. Adjust the flavor with a portion of pepper and salt to your liking.

Peking Pork Chops - Slow-Cooked

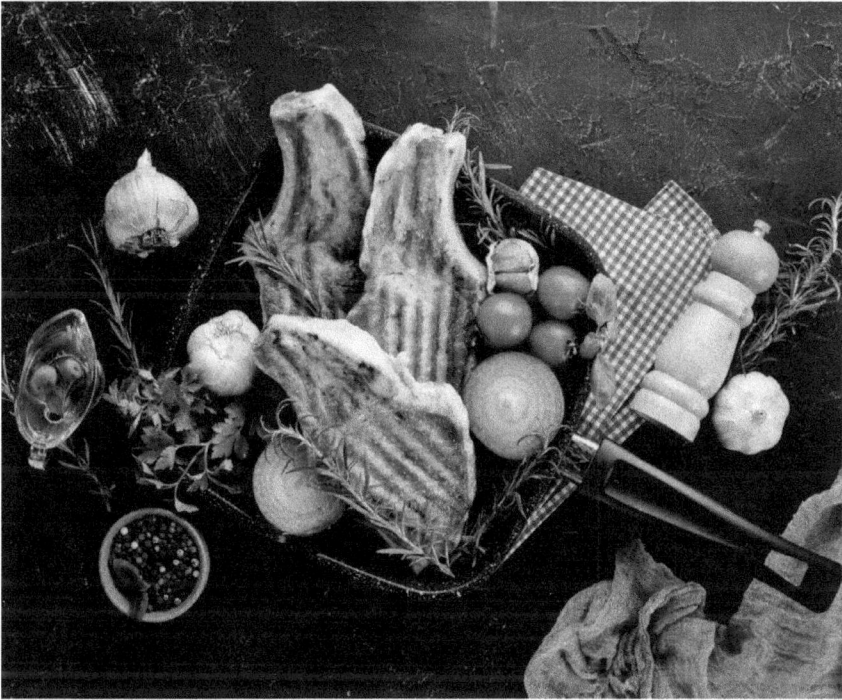

Servings Provided: 6

Time Required: 6 hours 15 minutes

What is Needed:

- Pork chops - top loin (6 boneless)
- Brown sugars (.25 cup)

- Ground ginger (1 tsp.)
- Shoyu soy sauce (.5 cup)
- Ketchup (.25 cup)
- Garlic (1 clove)
- Salt (as desired)

Preparation Method:

1. Use a sharp knife to remove the fat from the chops and toss them into the cooker.
2. Whisk the sugar, soy sauce, ginger, garlic, pepper, and salt. Dump it over the meat
3. Securely close the lid and set the timer for four to six hours.
4. Serve when it's tender with a dusting of salt and pepper as desired.

Chapter 5: Other Chinese Dishes

Crispy Tofu With Sweet & Sour Sauce

Servings Provided: 4

Time Required: 45 minutes

What is Needed:

The Sauce:

- Cornstarch (2 tsp.) + Water (2 tsp.)
- Garlic (2 minced cloves)
- Freshly grated ginger (.5 tsp.)
- Chili pepper flakes (.25 tsp.)
- Vegetable oil (2 tsp.)
- Water (.5 cup)
- Unseasoned rice vinegar (.33 cup)
- Agave nectar (.5 cup)
- Low-sodium soy sauce (2 tbsp.)
- Tomato paste (2 tbsp.)
- Sea salt (.25 tsp.)

The Tofu & Batter:

- Medium/firm tofu (1 brick)

- For Frying: Vegetable oil (3 cups)
- Cornstarch (1 tbsp.)
- Brown rice flour (1 cup)
- Ground pepper (.25 tsp.)
- Sea salt (.5 tsp.)
- Garlic powder (.5 tsp.)
- Cold soda water (1 cup)

Preparation Method:

1. Drain the brick of tofu and chop it into bite-sized cubes. Continue to drain the cubes on a layer of paper towels to remove the excess water. Press it often while you prepare the sauce.
2. Mix water with the cornstarch in a cup and set it aside for now.
3. Warm two teaspoons of vegetable oil using the med-low temperature setting. Mince and add the ginger, garlic, and chili pepper flakes. Stir for 30 seconds to one minute until fragrant.
4. Whisk in the rest of the sauce ingredients using the medium setting until it's bubbly. Whisk in the cornstarch mixture.
5. Whisk the sauce often for 10-12 minutes until slightly thickened. Transfer the pan to a cool burner while you prepare the crispy tofu.
6. Warm three cups of oil in an electric skillet or pan to reach 375° Fahrenheit.
7. Mix the batter by combining the rice flour, cornstarch, sea salt, garlic powder, and ground pepper in a mixing container.
8. When the pan is hot, stir in the soda water to the flour mixture and

mix well.

9. Use your hands to coat three to four cubes of tofu and gently place them into the oil. Fry them for 2-2.5 minutes.

10. Remove the tofu using a slotted spoon and place them onto a layer of paper towels to absorb the excess fat. Repeat the process with the rest of the tofu cubes.

11. Warm the sauce if needed. In two to three batches, you can coat the crispy tofu with sauce by adding a portion of the sauce to a large bowl and tossing the crispy tofu cubes until coated evenly. Serve to your liking with veggies or rice.

Shiitake & Scallion Lo Mein

Servings Provided: 8

Time Required: 40 minutes

What is Needed:

- Lo mein noodles (1 lb.)
- Snow peas (.25 lb.)
- Mirin (.25 cup)
- Soy sauce (.25 cup)
- Toasted sesame oil (2 tsp.)
- Canola oil (3 tbsp.)
- Shiitake mushrooms (1 lb.)
- Scallions (6)
- Fresh ginger (1 tbsp.)
- Water (2 tbsp.)
- Cilantro (2 tbsp.)

Preparation Method:

1. Slice the snow peas diagonally into halves. Remove the stems and thinly slice the caps of the mushrooms. Cut the scallions into one-inch lengths. Mince the ginger and chop the cilantro.

2. Prepare a large pot of boiling salted water. Cook the noodles until tender, adding in the snow peas for the last two minutes of the cooking cycle. Rinse and drain the noodles and snow peas in a colander using cold water until cooled.

3. Whisk the soy sauce with the sesame oil and mirin.

4. Prep a deep skillet to warm two tablespoons of the canola oil until shimmering using the high-temperature setting. Add the shiitake and cook it, undisturbed, until browned (5 min.).

5. Add the rest of the canola oil, scallions, and ginger. Stir-fry until the scallions softened (3 min.).

6. Add the water into the pan and simmer using moderate heat, scraping up the browned bits from the bottom of the pan for about a minute or so.

7. Mix in the snow peas, noodles, and soy sauce mixture. Simmer while tossing the noodles until they are thoroughly heated (2 min.).

8. Sprinkle using the cilantro and transfer it onto banana leaf cones or bowls to serve.

www.ingramcontent.com/pod-product-compliance
Lightning Source LLC
Chambersburg PA
CBHW060318030426
42336CB00011B/1099